ALZHEIMER'S DISEASE AND RELATED DISORDERS ANNUAL 5

ALZHEIMER'S DISEASE AND RELATED DISORDERS ANNUAL 5

Edited by

Serge Gauthier, MD FRCPC

Professor and Director
Alzheimer's Disease Research Unit
McGill Centre for Studies in Aging
Douglas Hospital
Verdun PQ
CANADA

Philip Scheltens, MD PhD

Department of Neurology / Alzheimer Center
Academisch Ziekenhuis
Vrije Universiteit
Amsterdam
The Netherlands

Jeffrey L Cummings, MD

Reed Neurological Research Center
University of California, Los Angeles
Los Angeles, CA
USA

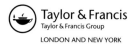

Taylor & Francis
Taylor & Francis Group

LONDON AND NEW YORK

© 2006 Taylor & Francis, an imprint of the Taylor & Francis Group

First published in the United Kingdom in 2006 by Taylor & Francis, an imprint of the Taylor & Francis Group, 2 Park Square, Milton Park, Abingdon, Oxon OX14 4RN

Tel.:   +44 (0)20 7017 6000
Fax.:   +44 (0)20 7017 6699
E-mail: info.medicine@tandf.co.uk
Website: www.tandf.co.uk/medicine

Although every effort has been made to ensure that all owners of copyright material have been acknowledged in this publication, we would be glad to acknowledge in subsequent reprints or editions any omissions brought to our attention.

Although every effort has been made to ensure that drug doses and other information are present- ed accurately in this publication, the ultimate responsibility rests with the prescribing physician. Neither the publishers nor the authors can be held responsible for errors or for any consequences arising from the use of information contained herein. For detailed prescribing information or instructions on the use of any product or procedure discussed herein, please consult the prescrib- ing information or instructional material issued by the manufacturer.

A CIP record for this book is available from the British Library.

Library of Congress Cataloging-in-Publication Data

Data available on application

ISBN 1 84184 561 2
      978 1 84184 561 6

Distributed in North and South America by

Taylor & Francis
2000 NW Corporate Blvd
Boca Raton, FL 33431, USA

Within Continental USA	Distributed in the rest of the world by
Tel: 800 272 7737;	Thomson Publishing Services
Fax: 800 374 3401	Cheriton House
Outside Continental USA	North Way
Tel: 561 994 0555;	Andover, Hampshire SP10 5BE, UK
Fax: 561 361 6018	Tel: +44 (0)1264 332424
E-mail: orders@crcpress.com	E-mail: salesorder.tandf@thomsonpublishingservices.co.uk

Composition by Creative
Printed and bound in Great Britain by TJ International Ltd, Padstow, Cornwall

Contents

Contributors

Charles Adler PhD
Mayo Clinic
Scottsdale, AZ
USA

Paul S Aisen MD
Department of Neurology
Georgetown University Medical Center
Washington, DC
USA

Laura D Baker PhD
Assistant Professor of Psychiatry and
Behavioral Sciences, University of
Washington School of Medicine,
Geriatric Research, Education and
Clinical Center, Veterans Affairs Puget
Sound Health Care System
Seattle, WA
USA

David A Bennett MD
Rush Alzheimer's Disease Center
Rush university Medical Center
Chicago, IL
USA

Lesley M Blake MD
Division of Geriatric Psychiatry
Northwestern University Medical
School
Chicago, IL
USA

Julie A Bobholz PhD
Assistant Professor of Neurology
Medical College of Wisconsin
Milwaukee, WI
USA

Patrick Browne MD
Center for Chest Disease
Division of Cardiology
Boswell Hospital
Sun City, AZ
USA

Donald Connor PhD
Cleo Roberts Clinical Research Center
Sun Health Research Institute
Sun City, AZ
USA

Suzanne Craft PhD
Professor of Psychiatry and Behavioral
Sciences
University of Washington School of
Medicine
Associate Director,
Geriatric Research, Education and
Clinical Center
Veterans Affairs Puget Sound Health
Care System
Seattle, WA
USA

Jeffrey L Cummings MD
Department of Neurology
David Geffen School of Medicine at
UCLA
Los Angeles, CA
USA

Kathryn Davis BA
Sun Health Research Institute
Sun City, AZ
USA

Steven T DeKosky MD
Department of Neurology
University of Pittsburgh School of
Medicine
Pittsburgh, PA
USA

FE De Leeuw MD PhD
Department of Neurology
University Medical Center St. Radboud
Nijmegen
The Netherlands

Mony de Leon PhD
New York University School of
Medicine
Center for Brain Health
New York, NY
USA

Murat Emre MD
Professor of Neurology
Head, Behavioral Neurology and
Movement Disorders Unit
Department of Neurology
Istanbul Faculty of Medicine
Çapa, Istanbul
Turkey

Denis Garceau PhD
Drug Development
Neurochem
Laval, Quebec
Canada

Serge Gauthier MD FRCPC
Professor and Director
Alzheimer's Disease Research Unit
McGill Centre for Studies in Aging
Douglas Hospital
Verdun PQ
Canada

Francine Gervais PhD
Vice-President, R&D
Neurochem
Laval
Quebec
Canada

Angela Gleason PhD
Postdoctoral Fellow
Department of Neurology
Medical College of Wisconsin
Milwaukee, WI
USA

Ronald L Hamilton MD
Division of Neuropathology
Department of Pathology
University of Pittsburgh School of
Medicine
Pittsburgh, PA
USA

Harald Hampel PhD
Department of Psychiatry
University of Munich
Nussbaumstr. 7
Munich
Germany

Milos D Ikonomovic MD
Alzheimer's Disease Research Center
University of Pittsburgh School of
Medicine
Pittsburgh, PA
USA

Sherry Johnson-Traver
Sun Health Research Institute
Sun City, AZ
USA

Raj N Kalaria MD
Wolfson Research Centre
Institute for Ageing and Health
Newcastle General Hospital
Westgate Road
Newcastle upon Tyne
UK

Jeff Lochhead BS
Sun Health Research Institute
Sun City, AZ
USA

Jean Lopez RN MSN
Cleo Roberts Clinical Research Center
Sun Health Research Institute
Sun City, AZ
USA

Jacobo E Mintzer MD
Medical University of South Carolina
Charleston, SC
USA

Elliot J Mufson PhD
Division of Neuroscience
Rush University
Rush Presbyterian St Luke's Medical
Center
Chicago, IL
USA

Suzana Petanceska PhD
Nathan Kline Institute and
Deptartments of Psychiatry and
Pharmmacology
New York University Medical Center
Orangeburg, NY
USA

Mark A Reger PhD
Acting Assistant Professor of Psychiatry
and Behavioral Sciences
University of Washington School of
Medicine
Geriatric Research, Education and
Clinical Center
Veterans Affairs Puget Sound Health
Care System
Seattle, WA
USA

Donald R Royall MD
Julia and Van Buren Parr Professor
for Alzheimer's research in psychiatry
Chief: Geriatric Psychiatry Division
The University of Texas Health Sciences
Center at San Antonio
San Antonio, TX
USA

Marwan Sabbagh MD
Cleo Roberts Clinical Research Center
Sun Health Research Institute
Sun City, AZ
USA

Philip Scheltens MD PhD
Department of Neurology/Alzheimer
Center
VU University Medical Center
Amsterdam
The Netherlands

Niki Schoonenboom MD
Department of Neurology/Alzheimer
Center
VU University Medical Center
Amsterdam
The Netherlands

Nina Silverberg PhD
Sun Health Research Institute
Sun City, AZ
USA

Holly Soares PhD
Pfizer Global R&D
Groton, CT
USA

D Larry Sparks PhD
Ralph and Muriel Roberts Laboratory
for Neurodegenerative Disease Research
and
The Cleo Roberts Center for Clinical
Research
Sun Health Research Institute
Sun City, AZ
USA

Cornelis J Stam MD PhD
Professor of Clinical Neurophysiology
Department of Clinical
Neurophysiology
VU University Medical Center
Amsterdam
The Netherlands

Suhair Stipho-Majeed MB ChB
CCRC
Sun Health Research Institute
Sun City, AZ
USA

Paul Volodarsky BS
Sun Health Research Institute
Sun City, AZ
USA

David Wilkinson MD
Consultant in Old Age Psychiatry and
Honorary Clinical Senior Lecturer
Memory Assessment and Research
Centre
Moorgreen Hospital
Botley Road
West End
Southampton
UK

Chuck Ziolkowski BS
Sun Health Research Institute
Sun City, AZ
USA

1
Neuropathology of mild cognitive impairment in the elderly

Steven T DeKosky, Milos D Ikonomovic, Ronald L Hamilton,
David A Bennett, and Elliot J Mufson

INTRODUCTION

The relationship of neuropathologic changes to the clinical status of people
with dementia is of paramount importance in devising appropriate therapeutic
interventions. Despite the fact that a central feature of the diagnostic criteria
for Alzheimer's disease (AD) includes a history of insidious onset and a progression of cognitive decline, it was not until the mid 1990s, as large-scale
memory clinics obtained increased experience with people presenting early
with symptoms of mild dementia, that attention was directed at understanding
the processes occurring during the prodromal stages of dementia. Subsequently, individuals with mild memory loss, who were clinically followed
as their cognition deteriorated through stages of mild, moderate, and
severe AD, were neuropathologically confirmed postmortem as AD. These
neuropathologic findings, together with retrospective and prospective imaging
studies, led to a reexamination of our concepts of the neuropathologic changes
underlying the onset of early symptoms of cognitive impairment, as well as
the clinical definition of prodromal AD. Because it is believed that AD has an
extensive preclinical phase, it is important to identify people in an early stage
when brain pathology has been initiated but prior to significant clinical symptoms. During the past few years, the concept of mild cognitive impairment
(MCI) has developed as a possible prodromal stage of AD. Although the precise definition of MCI is being debated, recent evidence suggests that MCI falls
into several subtypes. Individuals with isolated memory loss, termed amnestic
mild cognitive impairment (aMCI), represent the most extensively analyzed
form of MCI in specialty clinics. The 'conversion rate' of aMCI people to AD
(the time at which they meet current formal criteria for AD) is 10–15% annu-
ally.[1] On the other hand, mild impairment defined by deficits in other cognitive (and functional) domains is termed multiple domain MCI (mdMCI) and
may also occur as memory function declines below a defined threshold. In a
recent series of studies examining the onset of MCI in the Cardiovascular
Health Study (CHS) cohort, the risk factors for developing MCI included
apoE4 genotype (for aMCI), depression, racial and constitutional factors, and

the presence of cerebrovascular disease.[2] In this population-based study, about two-thirds of the MCI cases were mdMCI, and about one-third were aMCI.[3] Thus, a MCI is not as common in population-studies, and may be a less frequent manner of progressing to AD. This chapter provides an overview of neurobiologic observations crucial to our understanding of the chemical, pathologic, and molecular changes which occur in brain during the transitional period between normal aging and the clinical diagnosis of all forms of MCI and AD.

CLINICAL PRESENTATION OF MILD COGNITIVE IMPAIRMENT

Clinical and neuropathologic data necessary for the investigation of MCI have been derived from two types of cohorts. First are large clinic populations, which have (small numbers of) subjects who come to autopsy while still clinically classified as MCI. For example, the Alzheimer Disease Center at Washington University, St Louis, have reported autopsy results from their cohort of cases, some of whom died with a Clinical Dementia Rating (CDR) of 0.5, indicative of MCI.[4,5] A second source are volunteer cohorts of individuals in a population study, such as the Nun Study[6] and the Religious Orders Study (ROS),[7,8] in which all subjects agree to yearly cognitive and neurologic examination and brain autopsy at time of death. Because of their large size and advanced age of their subjects, these cohorts enable the assessment of the extent of pathologic and neurochemical changes in the brain associated with cognitive changes in particular diagnostic categories, including normal cognition, MCI, and mild, moderate, and severe AD. In all of these cohorts MCI marked a transitional state, with a decline of cognitive function that exceeded the norms for the respective populations. However, the definitions of MCI were somewhat different across cohorts. For example, a 0.5 CDR is used by several groups as an indicator of MCI, whereas the ROS uses an actuarial decision tree that incorporates and can be overridden by clinical judgment, and the Nun Study employs neuropsychologic testing patterns. Thus, the clinical definition or diagnosis of MCI remains variable and perhaps controversial. In this regard, Washington University utilized the CDR scale[9,10] to determine the presence or absence of MCI (CDR 0.5) and referred to them either as very mild AD or 'early stage AD'.[11] Because the CDR 0.5 represents a global cognitive score, these studies were careful in characterizing the specific cognitive domains that can be affected in MCI subjects, segregating them further into groups where cognitive impairment is uncertain (CDR 0.5/uncertain dementia), or detected selectively in the memory domain (CDR 0.5), in memory and up to two other domains (CDR 0.5/incipient dementia of the Alzheimer's type, DAT), or in memory and no less than 3 CDR domains (CDR 0.5/DAT).[11] Less confident diagnosis of MCI was categorized as CDR 0/0.5, which proved not to be distinct neuropathologically from CDR 0.5.[5,12] The CDR 0.5 cases are comparable to MCI subjects from the ROS cohort or to 'mild impairment – memory impaired' subjects from the Nun Study.[6]

Clinical evaluation of the ROS population relied on a battery of tests that included MMSE (Mini-Mental State Examination) as a measure of global cognitive function,[13] seven tests of episodic memory, and 13 tests of other cognitive abilities (for details of the cognitive function tests in ROS, see Wilson et al[14]). Based on these tests, MCI subjects in the ROS were classified into aMCI with impaired episodic memory and non-amnestic MCI without episodic memory impairment.[15] In the Nun Study, MCI were defined as subjects without dementia, who had preserved global cognition (measured by MMSE) and normal daily activities, but who were impaired in either memory or another cognitive domain.[6] However, the authors recognized that their MCI subjects represented a mixed group of individuals impaired in multiple areas of cognition, or domains other than memory, whereas only a small proportion of them were impaired in the isolated memory domain.[6] Similarly, many MCI cases in the ROS studies are most likely also mdMCI, with impairment in one or more cognitive areas.

Amyloid plaque pathology in MCI

The neuropathology of MCI is now being investigated in large-scale studies. Studies from Washington University in St Louis have provided evidence that virtually all subjects with a CDR score of 0.5 (approximately equivalent to aMCI) displayed sufficient numbers of amyloid beta (Aβ) plaques and neurofibrillary tangles (NFTs) to meet neuropathologic criteria for AD at autopsy.[11] Using Khachaturian pathologic criteria,[16] only 1 in 8 of those cases with no evidence of cognitive problems (CDR = 0 at entry and at death) showed neuropathologic evidence of AD. While this suggests that many MCI cases are preclinical AD, it did not define the extent of pathologic changes at the time the person was first diagnosed with MCI. Recent clinical pathologic investigations[17,18] provided evidence that 60% of MCI cases met the neuropathologic diagnosis of AD according to CERAD[19] and NIA-Reagan[20] criteria. Similarly, Petersen and colleagues reported that most of their MCI cases postmortem displayed significant neuropathologic changes similar to AD.[1] Given that AD (and MCI) are being diagnosed earlier and earlier in the progression of dementia, perhaps it is time to rethink whether the amounts of pathology needed to characterize a case as pathologic AD should be lower than allowed by the current diagnostic standards.

Despite the fact that Aβ plaques symbolize one of the major neuropathologic hallmarks of AD, their role in the initiation of AD dementia remains unclear. Neuropathologic studies of cognitively normal elderly have found that some already have considerable Aβ deposition in the brain.[5,21] More importantly, virtually all patients with MCI have Aβ plaques.[5,22–24] Because Aβ deposition is an early event in the course of AD, leading to other pathologies (e.g. synapse loss, neuronal degeneration, and NFT formation) which correlate more closely with cognitive decline,[25,26] it becomes increasingly important to define the extent of Aβ pathology during clinical changes from cognitively intact to MCI to AD.

Postmortem analysis of subjects in the St Louis community cohort found significant numbers of Aβ plaques in hippocampal and neocortical regions in both CDR 0.5 and CDR 0/0.5 subjects.[27,28] The CDR 0.5 are not easily distinguished from CDR 0/0.5 (questionable dementia), and were variably considered as MCI or 'early stage AD' or 'very mild dementia'.[11,27] The scarce pathology in cognitively normal (CDR 0) individuals, reported in these and other studies, indicates that brains of healthy aged people are, in general, spared from Aβ pathology and should be discriminated from 'pathologic aging'.[29] The CDR 0.5 cases had substantial and widespread Aβ plaques in the neocortex and to a lesser extent in the hippocampus, with a preponderance of the diffuse type in the neocortex, and of neuritic types in the limbic regions [5]. The pattern of Aβ plaque pathology across subjects with CDR 0 and CDR 0.5 led Price and colleagues to propose a continuum of Aβ plaque type that changes during the conversion from normal (scarce diffuse plaques) to pathologic aging and MCI or 'very mild dementia' (many diffuse and neuritic plaques).[12] The two clinical groups were different, based on densities of diffuse and neuritic Aβ plaques in the entorhinal cortex (ERC) and temporal neocortex,[22] supporting the theory that Aβ plaques may be of diagnostic value in MCI.[4,30]

The observations of extensive Aβ plaque pathology in MCI had been confirmed in other cohorts. The Baltimore Longitudinal Study of Aging[31] included two subjects with questionable dementia (CDR 0.5) who had moderate neuritic plaque frequencies, and were assigned neuropathologic diagnoses of probable AD. A clinical pathologic investigation of cases from the Jewish Home and Hospital in New York revealed that, compared with subjects with CDR 0, the CDR 0.5 subjects with questionable dementia had significantly increased densities of neuritic plaques in frontal, temporal, and parietal cortex, but not in occipital cortex, ERC, hippocampus, and amygdala.[23] These data further suggest that an increase in neocortical Aβ pathology parallels the earliest sign of cognitive decline in AD. An immunohistochemical study of Aβ load in the ERC from ROS subjects clinically diagnosed as MCI, not cognitively impaired (NCI), or mild to moderate AD found that the MCI cases were intermediate between the other two groups, with wide overlap and no statistically significant difference.[24] Aβ plaques were found in 83% of MCI, and the highest Aβ load measured in this study was in an MCI case with a neuropathologic diagnosis of possible AD. The wide range of Aβ content in subjects with MCI, and the considerable overlap with cognitively normal and demented subjects, further supported the suggestion of MCI as a transitional stage from normal aging to AD. Furthermore, this indicates that some MCI subjects resist deteriorating into dementia despite a considerable amount of plaque pathology in their mesial temporal lobe. Alternatively, it is possible that the addition of plaque pathology in other brain regions is more relevant for the clinical manifestation of dementia.

Biochemical measurements of $A\beta_{40}$ and $A\beta_{42}$

Neocortical tissue obtained postmortem from subjects selected from the Jewish Home and Hospital in New York was examined for soluble and insoluble $A\beta_{40}$ and $A\beta_{42}$ levels and revealed significant variability of total amyloid levels across CDR groups.[32] Compared to normal (CDR 0) controls, the CDR 0.5 subjects (questionable dementia) showed elevated levels of both $A\beta$ species in the ERC, frontal, parietal, and visual cortex, similar to the Washington University findings of increased $A\beta$ plaques in their CDR 0.5 cases, although curiously not in the temporal lobe. Elevation of both $A\beta_{40}$ and $A\beta_{42}$ levels correlated with the advancement of dementia. The authors concluded that elevations in $A\beta$ levels occurred very early in the disease progression, and this increase might influence the development of other types of AD pathology.

In cerebrospinal fluid (CSF) samples and magnetic resonance imaging (MRI) measurements taken from MCI and normal aged control subjects at baseline and 1 year later, deLeon and colleagues combined ventricular volume increases with measures of $A\beta$ as well as phosphorylated tau (pTau231).[33] Cross-sectionally, $A\beta_{40}$ but not $A\beta_{42}$ was increased, as was pTau231. One year later, the only significant change was an increase in pTau231, and that was only if the ventricular enlargement (implying greater CSF volume) was considered in the calculations.

Tau/neurofibrillary pathology in MCI

Unlike $A\beta$ plaques, which may not be present in the brains of some of the very elderly,[4] NFTs are an expected finding in all aged brains, although they may be few in number and restricted to the ERC or hippocampus.[34–38] Considerable amounts of pathologic tau (hyperphosphorylated tau aggregated into NFTs and neuropil threads) have been reported in MCI. Price and colleagues[4,5] showed that 'very mildly demented'/MCI cases (CDR 0/0.5 or 0.5) displayed increased numbers of NFTs, particularly in the ERC and perirhinal cortex, when compared with cognitively normal (CDR 0) controls. However, CDR 0 controls often display NFTs in the medial temporal structures. Whereas a subgroup of these NFT-positive CDR 0 cases lacked $A\beta$ deposits, in CDR 0.5 cases NFTs were always accompanied by $A\beta$ plaques, with the plaques being more abundant in neocortical areas.[5] It was suggested that the initial NFT pathology can occur without the presence of $A\beta$ plaques; however, advanced NFT densities are most likely to occur following $A\beta$ plaque formation.[5] In a review of their cases, Morris and Price[30] noted that NFT distribution in these very mild cases had not extended beyond the mesial temporal lobe, and suggested that the presence of diffuse $A\beta$ plaques in the cortex marked the onset of AD.

Examination of subjects from the Baltimore Longitudinal Study of Aging found that CDR 0.5 cases manifested NFTs in the hippocampus and amygdala, only scarce numbers of NFTs were seen in ERC or inferior parietal cortex,

whereas other neocortical regions lacked NFTs.[31] Similar findings were reported for CDR 0 controls in this study, consistent with observations by Price and
colleagues.[5] These observations suggest that, unlike Aβ plaques, NFTs are less
likely to aid the distinction between normal aging and MCI. However, there is
a dramatic increase in entorhinal/hippocampal NFTs in the CDR 0.5 compared
to CDR 0.[28]

Clinical pathologic investigations of subjects derived from the Jewish Home
and Hospital in New York revealed a significant positive correlation between
NFT densities and CDR scores.[37] However, NFT density in the CDR 0.5 subjects with 'questionable dementia' was not different from CDR 0 controls; both
groups had NFTs in the ERC and hippocampus. This study suggested that
NFT pathology increased with progression of dementia severity, but it was not
a reliable pathologic marker to distinguish MCI. Similarly, a study of
"oldest-old" subjects autopsied in the Geriatric Hospital of the University of
Geneva in Switzerland showed that Braak neuropathologic staging[39] correlated
highly with clinical CDR scores. However, it was difficult to distinguish
between CDR 0 and CDR 0.5 groups in this cohort.[38]

In the ROS population, the status of tau pathology was examined in MCI
(MMSE 26.8 ± 2, not different from controls), mild to moderate AD, and aged
control cases.[40] This study reported correlation of granulovacuolar and fibrillar lesions with several measures of episodic memory. Neuropil threads (NT)
preceded the appearance of NFT, which in turn appeared prior to neuritic Aβ
plaques. There were no statistically significant correlations between tau
pathology measurements and clinical classifications of NCI, MCI, and AD. A
quantitative stereologic investigation of phosphorylated tau pathology in the
parahippocampal gyrus from MCI, NCI, and AD subjects from the ROS cohort
demonstrated that MCI (MMSE 25.8 ± 2.9, not different from NCI) had a non-
significant increase in both NFT and NT densities compared to NCI.[41] In
contrast, the AD subjects showed significantly increased NFTs compared to
controls, but not MCI, and were comparable to controls with respect to NT
pathology.[41] Increasing NFT (but not NT) pathology correlated with impaired
performance on a measurement of episodic memory, suggesting that NFT
pathology plays a role in the clinical progression from NCI to MCI, and further into AD. DeKosky and colleagues examined the relationship between the
extent of neuropathologic changes by NIA/Reagan criteria[18] or Braak stage[42]
and choline acetyltransferase (ChAT) activity levels in ROS subjects. Almost
half of the MCI group had intermediate likelihood (NIA/Reagan category) of
AD, with another 11% having high likelihood;[18] 53% of persons with MCI
were Braak stage III/IV and 18% were Braak stage V/VI.[42] These observations
of significant AD pathology in MCI were confirmed in an enlarged cohort of
MCI subjects from the same ROS cohort.[8]

Further support for the hypothesis that NFT pathology influences MCI is
derived from a clinical pathologic evaluation of brain tissue harvested from the
Nun Study. This study reported a strong correlation between the progression
of NFT pathology, as defined by Braak staging, and cognitive impairment,

especially in the younger age groups.[6] About half of MCI subjects (with intact or impaired memory) were Braak stage I/II. This investigation pointed out the variability of neuropathologic findings in mildly impaired people with or without memory problems, at different stages of cognitive impairment at time of death. After separating their MCI cases into a group with significant memory impairment and those without much memory impairment, it was found that 23% of the non-memory impaired had Braak scores of 0 (no entorhinal NFTs). On the other hand, in the memory impaired group, which is most comparable to MCI in the literature, no cases lacked NFTs in the entorhinal/transentorhinal area.

An investigation of participants in a longitudinal study at the University of Miami found that MCI patients (diagnosed as a selective impairment of memory function) showed considerably greater density of NFTs in the fusiform gyrus and medial temporal areas compared with non-demented controls, while Aβ plaques were variable.[43] Additional studies of the quantitative changes in tau pathology are needed to clarify whether this or other types of pathology play a role in the clinical symptoms of MCI. Definition of MCI needs to be carefully characterized in all such studies.

Neuronal cell pathology in MCI

Several studies have examined changes in neuronal numbers in MCI, focusing either on the mesial temporal cortex or the cholinergic basal forebrain nuclei (CBFN). The ERC, the major paralimbic cortical relay region for the transmission of cortical information to the hippocampus, was of interest because it undergoes neurodegenerative changes in the earliest stages of disease progression.[28,39,44–47] Cases from the Washington University cohort showed no significant decrease in numbers of Nissl-stained neurons or ERC volume with age in healthy non-demented individuals. Few or no differences were observed between the healthy controls and what was termed 'preclinical AD', or cases with normal cognition (CDR 0) but a good deal of accumulated plaques and tangles at autopsy.[12] However, neuronal numbers were significantly decreased in the ERC (35%; 50% of cells in lamina II) and hippocampal CA1 (46% loss) in very mild AD (CDR 0/0.5 or CDR 0.5); cell loss was even more profound in severe AD. These findings suggest that cell atrophy and death have already occurred at a time when patients begin to manifest clinical symptoms of AD. The results of these studies are consistent with a previous report by Gomez-Isla and colleagues using cases from Washington University, which showed similar neuronal loss in the ERC (32%; 57% in lamina II).[28] Unbiased quantitative stereology revealed significant loss of NeuN-immunoreactive neurons in the ERC lamina II of MCI (63%) and mild to moderate AD (58%) in cases derived from the ROS cohort.[47] Moreover, there was also a reduction in lamina II ERC volume in MCI (26%) and AD (43%), in agreement with previous findings.[12] ERC atrophy correlated with impairment on MMSE and clinical tests of declarative memory.[30,47]

Cholinergic basal forebrain system dysfunction

The cholinotrophic phenotype of the CBFN neurons is altered during the prodromal and earliest stages of AD. Quantitative stereologic studies revealed that
the number of nucleus basalis (NB) perikarya expressing either ChAT, the synthetic enzyme for acetylcholine, or the vesicular acetylcholine transporter
(VAChT) was stable in MCI and mild AD.[48] Moreover, other studies demonstrated that ChAT activity in NB cortical projection sites is unchanged in mild
AD.[17,18] Taken together, these observations suggest that the enzymes underlying basocortical cholinergic neurotransmission are preserved in MCI and early
AD, although cholinergic function is probably impaired as these neurons contain NFTs.[49] The number of NB perikarya expressing either the high-affinity
nerve growth factor (NGF)-selective receptor trkA or the pan-neurotrophin
receptor p75[NTR] was reduced ~50% in MCI and mild AD compared with NCI,
and this deficit correlated significantly with impaired performance on the
MMSE and a few individual tests of working memory and attention.[50,51] Many
cholinergic NB neurons appear to undergo a phenotypic silencing of NGF
receptor expression in the absence of frank neuronal loss during the early
stages of cognitive decline, as trkA (but not p75[NTR] mRNA) was reduced in
NB neurons in MCI and AD[52] as well as in the cortex.[53] These alterations may
signify an early deficit in neurotrophic support during the progression of AD:
perhaps this related to the early declines in cholinergic function and the
sensitivity of the cholinergic system to cholinergic blockers.[54]

NGF levels are preserved in the hippocampus and neocortex in MCI subjects.[55] ProNGF (the precursor molecule for NGF) is elevated 1.4 times above
controls in the parietal cortex in MCI, and 1.6 times above control levels in
mild AD.[56] Thus, the perturbations in NGF signaling within the cholinotrophic basal forebrain system in early AD may be initiated by defective NGF retrograde transport due to reduced receptor protein levels in cortical projection
sites, which ultimately affects NB neuronal survival, or due to alteration in the
ratio of cortical proNGF to trkA.[53] The presence of cell cycle proteins within
NB neurons in MCI and mild AD cases from the ROS cohort[57] suggests that
cortical NGF receptor imbalance may contribute to the selective vulnerability
of cholinergic NB neurons via deficits in trkA-mediated pro-survival signaling
and/or alterations in p75[NTR]-mediated signaling, which promotes unscheduled
cell cycle re-entry and apoptosis during the prodromal stages of AD.

Collectively, these data support the concept that MCI is associated with phenotypic changes (e.g. trkA, p75[NTR]), but not frank neuronal degeneration, in
the CBFN. Factors other than these particular markers of cholinergic neurons,
or dysfunction of other cell populations (e.g. ERC lamina II neurons), also
play a role in the differences in cognitive function.

Cholinergic enzyme changes in MCI

ChAT loss has been regarded as the hallmark neurotransmitter change in AD.
Most investigators have always presumed that loss of cholinergic function

underlies much of the short-term memory loss in AD, and probably in MCI as well. The observations that physostigmine and oral anticholinesterases have beneficial effects for patients with AD suggest that the cholinergic basal forebrain system is altered despite the absence of ChAT enzyme deficits in AD. In fact, a series of studies have shown that neocortical ChAT activity is preserved in MCI.[17,18,58,59] Thus, cholinergic enzyme deficits are probably not the primary cause of the memory loss in MCI, although these studies do not rule out other types of cholinergic dysfunction early in the disease course. On the other hand, DeKosky and colleagues found elevated ChAT activity in the hippocampus and frontal cortex of subjects with MCI.[18] These results suggested that cognitive deficits in MCI and early AD are not associated with ChAT reduction in the hippocampus, and that select components of the hippocampal and cortical cholinergic projection system are capable of compensatory responses during the early stages of dementia. Increased hippocampal and frontal cortex ChAT activity in MCI may be important in promoting biochemical stability, or compensating for neurodegenerative defects, which may delay the transition of these subjects to AD. Interestingly, hippocampal ChAT activity was increased selectively in those MCI cases scored as a Braak III/IV stage, suggesting that a compensatory up-regulation of ChAT occurs during the progression of entorhinal–hippocampal NFT pathology.[42] This cholinergic upregulation is reminiscent of the cholinergic axonal plasticity response in the hippocampus following denervation or loss of excitatory input from the ERC lamina II neurons observed in animal models of AD[60] as well as in AD brains.[61,62] This neuronal reorganization may account for the increase in ChAT activity observed in the MCI hippocampus, considering the fact that NFT changes involved most of the ERC lamina II neurons by the time these subjects developed MCI.[18,42] The reasons for the elevation of ChAT in frontal cortex in MCI is less clear, but is most probably also the result of cholinergic sprouting.

Acetylcholinesterase (AChE), the enzyme that hydrolyzes acetylcholine at the synapse, did not show decline in cortical areas until at least moderately severe levels of dementia were present.[17] Positron emission tomography (PET) studies, utilizing a ligand that labels AChE in vivo, suggested that there is only mild loss of AChE in MCI[63] and mild AD.[64] Notably, in the latter study the loss in AD was less than that in Parkinson's disease or Parkinson's dementia. The manner in which this cholinergic enzyme impacts cognitive decline in AD remains an area of great interest. Studies utilizing AChE PET ligands in large sample sizes can be expected to be undertaken in the future.

Other neurochemical markers

Levels of isoprostane, 8,12-iso-iPF2alpha-VI, a sensitive marker for in-vivo lipid peroxidation (and thus of degree of oxidative stress), are elevated in urine, blood, and CSF in AD, and correlate with cognitive and functional scores as well as CSF tau and amyloid concentrations.[65] To the extent that the MCI cases had an intermediate level of the isoprostane, this study may indicate the degree of oxidative stress in the pathologic processes in MCI brains. If confirmed, this method might have promise for diagnosis and as a biomarker for the level of oxidative stress in AD.

Soluble alpha-synuclein (α-syn), a heat-stable protein that plays an important role in neuronal plasticity, was significantly reduced in the frontal cortex in AD patients compared with MCI and NCI patients from the ROS cohort; there were no differences between MCI and NCI.[66] The immunoreactivity of α-syn correlated with MMSE score and a global neuropsychologic z-score. Similar results were found in a study examining the relation of Lewy bodies identified with α-syn antibodies in the substantia nigra, limbic system, and several neocortical regions in cases from the ROS.[8] About 10% of patients with MCI and those without cognitive impairment had Lewy bodies; by contrast, more than 20% of patients with dementia had Lewy bodies.

Both MCI and AD groups had markedly elevated expression of heme oxygenase-1 (HO-1, an indirect marker of oxidative stress) in the hippocampus and temporal neocortex.[67] Astroglial HO-1 immunoreactivity in the temporal cortex, but not hippocampus, correlated with the burden of neurofibrillary pathology. These data strengthen earlier observations suggesting that oxidative stress may be a very early event in the pathogenesis of AD.

Synapse counts in MCI

Evaluation of synapse numbers in biopsy-derived[68] and postmortem[69] tissue show a high correlation with cognitive impairment. Although there are no published studies on the status of synaptic integrity in MCI, a preliminary stereologic analysis of synapse counts in the hippocampus from ROS cases showed remarkable variability.[70] In MCI, the number of synapses in two regions of the hippocampus (CA1 and outer molecular layer of dentate gyrus) was reduced on average, and the synaptic densities seemed to fall either in the AD range or in the range of the controls. More cases will be needed to determine the precise nature of synapse loss in different regions of brain during the progression of AD.

Subcortical (white matter) changes and cerebrovascular disease

Subcortical white matter alterations and loss (subcortical atrophy leading to hydrocephalus ex vacuo) are well-known correlates of AD. Thus, age-related white matter changes, such as ubiquitin-immunoreactive granular degeneration of myelin, may occur during the progression of AD and contribute to cognitive (and motor) dysfunction. In an immunohistochemical study of ubiquitin and myelin basic protein (MBP) in frontal white matter of subjects from the ROS cohort, MBP was significantly decreased (28%) in mild AD but not in MCI compared with control brain white matter samples.[71] MBP changes correlated with both global and frontal function-specific tests of cognition, suggesting that white matter pathology may contribute to age- and disease-associated cognitive decline.

An examination of the relationship of macroscopic cerebral infarctions to MCI in ROS demonstrated that one-third of MCI cases had cerebral infarctions.[8] This was in contrast to nearly 50% of patients with dementia and less than 25% of patients without cognitive impairment.

CONCLUSIONS

Neuropathologic and neurochemical studies are emerging to aid in the definition of the brain's status during the earliest stages of symptomatic cognitive impairment as well as presymptomatic AD. Initial conclusions suggest that significant Aβ deposition, NFT formation, and neuronal cell loss (especially in the mesial temporal lobe), and alterations in the NGF neurotrophin receptor system, are evident, but without major differences between cases with a clinical diagnosis of MCI at death and those clinically diagnosed as 'mild' AD. Other significant markers, or system disruptions, are yet to be identified. In addition, the synaptic and cholinergic plasticity, which may differ from individual to individual, no doubt contribute to the variability of the pathologic findings. Based upon the multiple markers thus far explored, variability in the MCI cases is going to be multidimensional, and there is no indication that one specific pathologic or biochemical variable will be an absolute quantitative marker of MCI.

It does not appear possible to predict accurately the extent/severity of neuropathologic changes based only on the cognitive status of an individual. In cognitively normal cases with only small numbers of NFTs in the ERC and few or no Aβ deposits anywhere, one cannot accept these as being AD or even incipient AD. However, we can, to some degree, feel confident that nearly all cases with some cognitive impairment (even MCI) will show pathologic changes with varying degrees of NFTs and Aβ plaques. MCI cases have a range of AD pathology that includes NFTs in the ERC and Aβ deposits in the neocortex, and show considerable overlap with the pathology found in 'early AD' to such an extent that it is still impossible in a given case to accurately predict the severity of clinical impairment based on the neuropathologic changes when they are in low Braak stages (≤stage III) and contain less than a moderate number of neuritic plaques in the neocortex.

There are several possible reasons for inconsistencies in the literature describing the neuropathology of MCI, including insufficient sample size, neuropathologic heterogeneity within and across diagnostic groups, selection of the measure of pathologic changes, lack of a unified clinical definition of MCI, and the possibility that the cognitive status at the time of death may have progressed from the one that was determined during the last neuropsychologic testing which served to establish the 'final' clinical diagnosis of MCI. Thus, the antemortem interval from the last clinical diagnosis to death needs to be as short as possible. In most of the studies presented in this chapter, the last clinical evaluation was performed within 1 year of death. A unified clinical diagnostic and neuropathologic testing procedure, which would serve for more consistent correlative investigations of cognitive status vs neuropathologic changes, would also be of immense benefit for MCI research. For a variety of logistical reasons, that is not likely to happen. However, agreement among groups which use different approaches would be powerful. The neuropathologic distinction between MCI and cognitively normal aged people, or those with early dementia, has also been difficult because a wide range of neuropathologic changes were present in each of these clinical diagnostic groups, with significant overlap. Brains of cognitively normal people often contain substantial amounts of neuropathologic changes, including Aβ plaques and NFTs,[24,72,73] similar to what is seen in MCI. Studies relying on quantitative biochemical measurements or direct (stereological) counting of neuropathologic changes might be of help in improving the clinical/pathologic correlates.

The search for the status of the brain in MCI will continue with postmortem analyses as well as in-vivo studies. Recent results indicate that Aβ imaging in vivo can be accomplished in AD.[74] Preliminary data on cases with MCI suggest that, like the synapse data, the means of Aβ load are midway between AD cases and controls, but that the individual cases lie either in the range of normals or in the range of AD cases. On the other hand, recent MRI studies indicate that MCI have reduced ERC and hippocampal volume[75,76] and higher rate of hippocampal volume loss.[77] It is unlikely that a single marker, neuropathologic or clinical, will emerge as a standard measure of MCI-specific pathology. However, since there is great neuropathology overlap between MCI and AD, the current data suggest that MCI is a prodromal form of AD.

ACKNOWLEDGMENTS

This work was supported by the NIA grants AG05133, AG14449, AG16668, AG09446 and AG10161.

REFERENCES

1. Petersen R. Mild Cognitive Impairment: Aging to Alzheimer's Disease. New York: Oxford University Press, 2003.

2. Lopez OL, Jagust WJ, Dulberg C, et al. Risk factors for mild cognitive impairment in the Cardiovascular Health Study Cognition Study: part 2. Arch Neurol 2003;60:1394–1399.

3. Lopez OL, Jagust WJ, DeKosky ST, et al. Prevalence and classification of mild cognitive impairment in the Cardiovascular Health Study Cognition Study: part 1. Arch Neurol 2003;60:1385–1389.

4. Price JL, Davis PD, Morris JC, et al. The distribution of tangles, plaques and related immunohistochemical

markers in healthy aging and Alzheimer's disease. Neurobiol Aging 1991;12:295–312.

5. Price JL, Morris JC. Tangles and plaques in nondemented aging and "preclinical" Alzheimer's disease. Ann Neurol 1999;45:358–368.

6. Riley KP, Snowdon DA, Markesbery WR. Alzheimer's neurofibrillary pathology and the spectrum of cognitive function: findings from the Nun Study. Ann Neurol 2002; 51:567–577.

7. Bennett DA, Wilson RS, Schneider JA, et al. Natural history of mild cognitive impairment in older persons. Neurology 2002;59:198–205.

8. Bennett DA, Schneider JA, Bienias JL, et al. Mild cognitive impairment is related to Alzheimer disease pathology and cerebral infarctions. Neurology 2005;64:834–841.

9. Hughes CP. A new clinical scale for staging of dementia. Br J Psychiatry 1982;140:566–572.

10. Morris JC. The Clinical Dementia Rating (CDR): current version and scoring rules. Neurology 1993;43: 2412–2413.

11. Morris JC, Storandt M, Miller JP, et al. Mild cognitive impairment represents early-stage Alzheimer disease. Arch Neurol 2001;58: 397–405.

12. Price JL, Ko AI, Wade MJ, et al. Neuron number in the entorhinal cortex and CA1 in preclinical Alzheimer's disease. Arch Neurol 2001;58:1395–1402.

13. Folstein MF, Folstein SE, McHugh PR. "Mini-mental state". A practical method grading the cognitive state of patients for the clinician. J Psychiatry Res 1975;12:189–198.

14. Wilson RS, Beckett LA, Barnes LL, et al. Individual differences in rates of change in cognitive abilities of older persons. Psychol Aging 2002;17: 179–193.

15. Aggarwal NT, Wilson RS, Beck TL, et al. The apolipoprotein E epsilon-4 allele and incident Alzheimer's disease in person's with mild cognitive impairment. Neurocase 2005;11:3–7.

16. Khachaturian ZS. Diagnosis of Alzheimer's disease. Arch Neurol 1985;42:1097–1105.

17. Davis KL, Mohs RC, Marin D, et al. Cholinergic markers in elderly patients with early signs of Alzheimer's disease. JAMA 1999; 281:1401–1406.

18. DeKosky ST, Ikonomovic MD, Styren S, et al. Upregulation of choline acetyltransferase activity in hippocampus and frontal cortex of elderly subjects with mild cognitive impairment. Ann Neurol 2002;51: 145–155.

19. Mirra SS, Heyman A, McKeel D, et al. The Consortium to Establish a Registry for Alzheimer's Disease (CERAD). Part II. Standardization of the neuropathologic assessment of Alzheimer's disease. Neurology 1991; 41:479–486.

20. National Institute on Aging and Reagan Institute working group on diagnosis criteria for the neuropathological assessment of Alzheimer's disease. Consensus recommendations for the postmortem diagnosis of AD. Neurobiol Aging 1997;18:S1–S3.

21. Braak H, Braak E. Frequency of stages of Alzheimer-related lesions in different age categories. Neurobiol Aging 1997;18:351–357.

22. Morris JC, Storandt M, McKeel DW, et al. Cerebral amyloid deposition and diffuse plaques in "normal" aging: evidence for presymptomatic and very mild Alzheimer's disease. Neurology 1996;44:707–719.

23. Haroutunian V, Perl DP, Purohit DP, et al. Regional distribution of neuritic plaques in the nondemented elderly and subjects with very mild Alzheimer disease. Arch Neurol 1998;55:1185–1191.

24. Mufson EJ, Chen EY, Cochran EJ, et al. Entorhinal cortex beta-amyloid load in individuals with mild cognitive impairment. Exp Neurol 1999;158:469–490.

25. Ingelsson M, Fukumoto H, Newell KL, et al. Early Abeta accumulation and progressive synaptic loss, gliosis, and tangle formation in AD brain. Neurology 2004;62:925–931.

26. Bennett DA, Schneider JA, Wilson RS, et al. Neurofibrillary tangles mediate the association of amyloid load with clinical Alzheimer disease and level of cognitive function. Arch Neurol 2004;61:378–384.

27. Morris JC, McKeel DW Jr, Storandt M, et al. Very mild Alzheimer's disease: informant-based clinical, psychometric, and pathologic distinction from normal aging. Neurology 1991;41:469–478.

28. Gomez-Isla T, Price JL, McKeel DW Jr, et al. Profound loss of layer II entorhinal cortex neurons occurs in very mild Alzheimer's disease. J Neurosci 1996;16:4491–4500.

29. Dickson DW, Crystal HA, Mattiace LA, et al. Identification of normal and pathological aging in prospectively studied nondemented elderly humans. Neurobiol Aging 1992;13:179–189.

30. Morris JC, Price AL. Pathologic correlates of nondemented aging, mild cognitive impairment, and early-stage Alzheimer's disease. J Mol Neurosci 2001;17:101–118.

31. Troncoso JC, Martin LJ, Dal Forno G, et al. Neuropathology in controls and demented subjects from the Baltimore Longitudinal Study of Aging. Neurobiol Aging 1996;17:365–371.

32. Naslund J, Haroutunian V, Mohs R, et al. Correlation between elevated levels of amyloid β-peptide in the brain and cognitive decline. JAMA 2000;283:1571–1577.

33. de Leon MJ, DeSanti S, Zinkowski R, et al. MRI and CSF studies in the early diagnosis of Alzheimer's disease. J Intern Med 2004;256:205–223.

34. Blessed G, Tomlinson B, Roth M. The association between quantitative measures of dementia and of senile changes in cerebral grey matter of elderly subjects. Br J Psychiatry 1968;114:797–811.

35. Tomlinson B, Blessed G, Roth M. Observations on the brains of demented old people. J Neurol Sci 1970;11:205–242.

36. Braak H, Braak E. Evolution of the neuropathology of Alzheimer's disease. Acta Neurol Scand Suppl 1996;165:3–12.

37. Haroutunian V, Purohit DP, Perl DP, et al. Neurofibrillary tangles in nondemented elderly subjects and mild Alzheimer disease. Arch Neurol 1999;56:713–718.

38. Gold G, Bouras C, Kovari E, et al. Clinical validity of Braak neuropathological staging in the oldest-old. Acta Neuropathol (Berl) 2000;99:579–582.

39. Braak H, Braak E. Neuropathological staging of Alzheimer's disease. Acta Neuropath 1991;82:239–259.

40. Ghoshal N, Garcia-Sierra F, Wuu J, et al. Tau conformational changes correspond to impairments of episodic memory in mild cognitive impairment and Alzheimer's disease. Exp Neurol 2002;177:475–493.

41. Mitchell TW, Mufson EJ, Schneider JA, et al. Parahippocampal tau pathology in healthy aging, mild cognitive impairment, and early Alzheimer's disease. Ann Neurol 2002;51:182–189.

42. Ikonomovic MD, Mufson EJ, Woo J, et al. Cholinergic plasticity in hippocampus of individuals with mild cognitive impairment: correlation with Alzheimer's neuropathology. J Alzheimers Disease 2003;5:39–48.

43. Guillozet AL, Weintraub S, Mash DC, et al. Neurofibrillary tangles, amyloid, and memory in aging and mild

cognitive impairment. Arch Neurol 2003;60:729–736.

44. Delacourte A, David JP, Sergeant N, et al. The biochemical pathway of neurofibrillary degeneration in aging and Alzheimer's disease. Neurology 1999;52:1158–1165.

45. Hyman BT, Van Hoesen GW, Damasio AR, et al. Alzheimer's disease: cell-specific pathology isolates the hippocampal formation. Science 1984;225:1168–1170.

46. Hyman B, Van Hoesen G, Kromer L, et al. Perforant pathway changes and memory impairment of Alzheimer's disease. Ann Neurol 1986;20: 472–481.

47. Kordower JH, Chu Y, Stebbins GT, et al. Loss and atrophy of layer II entorhinal cortex neurons in elderly people with mild cognitive impairment. Ann Neurol 2001;49:202–213.

48. Gilmor ML, Erickson JD, Varoqui H, et al. Preservation of nucleus basalis neurons containing choline acetyltransferase and the vesicular acetylcholine transporter in the elderly with mild cognitive impairment and early Alzheimer's disease. J Comp Neurol 1999;411:693–704.

49. Mesulam M, Shaw P, Mash D, et al. Cholinergic nucleus basalis tauopathy emerges early in the aging-MCI-AD continuum. Ann Neurol 2004;55:815–828.

50. Mufson EJ, Ma SY, Cochran EJ, et al. Loss of nucleus basalis neurons containing trkA immunoreactivity in individuals with mild cognitive impairment and early Alzheimer's disease. J Comp Neurol 2000;427: 19–30.

51. Mufson EJ, Ma SY, Dills J, et al. Loss of basal forebrain P75(NTR) immunoreactivity in subjects with mild cognitive impairment and Alzheimer's disease. J Comp Neurol 2002;443:136–153.

52. Chu Y, Cochran EJ, Beckett LA, et al. Down-regulation of trkA mRNA within nucleus basalis neurons in individuals with mild cognitive impairment and Alzheimer's disease. J Comp Neurol 2001;437: 296–307.

53. Counts SE, Nadeem M, Wuu J, et al. Reduction of cortical TrkA but not p75(NTR) protein in early-stage Alzheimer's disease. Ann Neurol 2004;56:520–531.

54. Sunderland T, Esposito G, Molchan SE, et al. Differential cholinergic regulation in Alzheimer's patients compared to controls following chronic blockade with scopolamine: a SPECT study. Psychopharmacology (Berl) 1995;121:231–241.

55. Mufson EJ, Ikonomovic MD, Styren SD, et al. Preservation of brain nerve growth factor in mild cognitive impairment and Alzheimer's disease. Arch Neurol 2003;60:1143–1148.

56. Peng S, Wuu J, Mufson EJ, et al. Increased proNGF levels in subjects with mild cognitive impairment and mild Alzheimer disease. J Neuropathol Exp Neurol 2004;63: 641–649.

57. Yang Y, Mufson EJ, Herrup K. Neuronal cell death is preceded by cell cycle events at all stages of Alzheimer's disease. J Neurosci 2003; 23:2557–2563.

58. Tiraboschi P, Hansen LA, Alford M, et al. The decline in synapses and cholinergic activity is asynchronous in Alzheimer's disease. Neurology 2000;55:1278–1283.

59. Ikonomovic MD, Mufson EJ, Wuu J, et al. Reduction of choline acetyltransferase activity in primary visual cortex in mild to moderate Alzheimer's disease. Arch Neurol 2005;62:425–430.

60. Cotman CW, Matthews DA, Taylor D, et al. Synaptic rearrangement in the dentate gyrus: Histochemical evidence of adjustments after lesions in immature and adult rats. Proc Natl Acad Sci USA 1973;70:3473–3477.

61. Geddes JW, Monaghan DT, Cotman CW, et al. Plasticity of hippocampal

circuitry in Alzheimer's disease. Science 1985;230:1179–1181.

62. Hyman BT, Kromer LJ, Van Hoesen GW. Reinnervation of the hippocampal perforant pathway zone in Alzheimer's disease. Ann Neurol 1987;21:259–267.

63. Rinne JO, Kaasinen V, Jarvenpaa T, et al. Brain acetylcholinesterase activity in mild cognitive impairment and early Alzheimer's disease. J Neurol Neurosurg Psychiatry 2003;74: 113–115.

64. Bohnen NI, Kaufer DI, Ivanco LS, et al. Cortical cholinergic function is more severely affected in parkinsonian dementia than in Alzheimer disease: an in vivo positron emission tomographic study. Arch Neurol 2003;60:1745–1748.

65. Pratico D, Clark CM, Lee VM, et al. Increased 8,12-iso-iPF2alpha-VI in Alzheimer's disease: correlation of a noninvasive index of lipid peroxidation with disease severity. Ann Neurol 2000;48:809–812.

66. Wang DS, Bennett DA, Mufson E, et al. Decreases in soluble alpha-synuclein in frontal cortex correlate with cognitive decline in the elderly. Neurosci Lett 2004;359:104–108.

67. Schipper HM, Bennett DA, Lieberman A, et al. Heme oxygenase-1 expression in MCI and early AD. Neurobiol Aging: in press.

68. DeKosky ST, Scheff SW. Synapse loss in frontal cortex biopsies in Alzheimer's disease: Correlation with cognitive severity. Ann Neurol 1990;27:457–464.

69. Terry RD, Masliah E, Salmon DP, et al. Physical basis of cognitive alterations in Alzheimer's disease: synapse loss is the major correlate of cognitive impairment. Ann Neurol 1991;30:572–580.

70. Scheff SW, Price DA, Schmitt FA, et al. Stereological assessment of hippocampal synapses in people with Alzheimer's disease and mild cognitive impairment. 9th Int. Conf. Alzheimer's Disease and Related Disorders 2004:3–170.

71. Wang DS, Bennett DA, Mufson EJ, et al. Contribution of changes in ubiquitin and myelin basic protein to age-related cognitive decline. Neurosci Res 2004;48:93–100.

72. Davis DG, Schmitt FA, Wekstein DR, et al. Alzheimer neuropathologic alterations in aged cognitively normal subjects. J Neuropath Exp Neurol 1999;58:376–388.

73. Knopman DS, Parisi JE, Salviati A, et al. Neuropathology of cognitively normal elderly. J Neuropath Exp Neurol 2003;62:1087–1095.

74. Klunk WE, Engler H, Nordberg A, et al. Imaging brain amyloid in Alzheimer's disease with Pittsburgh Compound-B. Ann Neurol 2004;55: 306–319.

75. Dickerson BC, Goncharova I, Sullivan MP, et al. MRI-derived entorhinal and hippocampal atrophy in incipient and very mild Alzheimer's disease. Neurobiol Aging 2001;22:747–754.

76. Du AT, Schuff N, Amend D, et al. Magnetic resonance imaging of the entorhinal cortex and hippocampus in mild cognitive impairment and Alzheimer's disease. J Neurol Neurosurg Psychiatry 2001;71: 441–447.

77. Jack CR Jr, Petersen RC, Xu Y, et al. Rates of hippocampal atrophy correlate with change in clinical status in aging and AD. Neurology 2000;55:484–489.

2

Cerebrospinal fluid markers for the diagnosis of Alzheimer's disease

Niki Schoonenboom, Harald Hampel, Philip Scheltens, and Mony de Leon

INTRODUCTION

Alzheimer's disease (AD) is considered to be the most common type of dementia.[1] Due to the aging of the population, the number of persons affected by AD is expected to increase three-fold by 2050.[2]

The diagnosis of AD is made by exclusion and based on clinical criteria,[3] supported by neuropsychologic tests, neuroimaging, and extended follow-up. In the early stage, it is difficult to differentiate AD from other types of dementia, as the clinical symptoms are subtle and the diagnostic methods may be normal. Furthermore, clinical overlap exists between the different types of dementias, while volume changes of the hippocampus and medial temporal lobe on magnetic resonance imaging (MRI) are not specific for AD.[4] With the advent of novel therapeutic strategies,[5] it became important to diagnose AD as early as possible, as pharmacologic treatment needs to be started before extensive and irreversible brain damage has occurred. Over the last decade, many studies have set out to find an appropriate biomarker for the diagnosis of AD.[6] This chapter starts with an overview as regards the most promising cerebrospinal fluid (CSF) biomarkers for the early and differential diagnosis of AD. Next, the relationship of the biomarkers and atrophy on MRI is discussed. Finally, limitations and topics for future research are presented.

Neuropathology

The basis for the research on biochemical markers are the neuropathologic changes present in the various types of dementias.[7] Neuropathologic hallmarks of AD – accumulation of extracellularly senile plaques (SPs) and neurofibrillary tangles (NFTs), synaptic reductions, and neuron loss – gradually accumulate in time, and start long before the clinical picture of AD becomes overt.[8] SPs are divided into two types: diffuse and neuritic plaques. The neuritic plaques are composed of the highly insoluble fibrillar protein amyloid β_{42} ($A\beta_{42}$). $A\beta$ depositions tend to accumulate with age. NFTs are intraneuronal accumulations of abnormally (hyper)phosphorylated tau protein. NFTs can be found already in non-demented subjects in the hippocampus and entorhinal cortex (EC), the regions affected earliest in AD. SPs are found initially in the neocortex, but in later stages they also affect the EC and the hippocampus.[9,10] Patients with frontotemporal dementia (FTD) show heterogeneity in underlying pathology,[11] with tau deposits in some of them. Creutzfeldt–Jakob disease (CJD) is characterized by spongiform changes, neuronal loss, gliosis and immunostaining of the protease-resistant prion protein.[12] Dementia with Lewy bodies (DLB) is part of the α-synucleinopathies, in which α-synuclein accumulates in the intraneuronal Lewy bodies.[13] Vascular dementia (VAD) is characterized by ischemic lesions, lacunes, and extensive white matter changes.[14] Between the different types of clinically diagnosed dementias significant neuropathologic overlap exists.[15] Lewy bodies are present in AD, whereas FTD, VAD and DLB plaques and tangles can be found. White matter changes are found in all types of dementia, especially in AD.[16]

CEREBROSPINAL FLUID AMYLOID β_{42} AND TAU IN ALZHEIMER'S DISEASE VS CONTROLS

According to criteria established in 1998, a good biomarker has to have a sensitivity of at least 85% for AD and a specificity of ≥75% to differentiate AD from other types of dementia.[7] The most promising CSF markers to differentiate AD from non-demented elderly are $A\beta_{42}$ and tau. Below, each biomarker is discussed separately. Next, the most valid studies will be summarized for the combination of CSF $A\beta_{42}$ and tau.

$A\beta_{42}$

In numerous studies it has been shown that $A\beta_{42}$ is decreased in CSF of AD patients compared with non-demented controls.[6,17] The decrease of $A\beta_{42}$ concentration in CSF is thought to be the result of several mechanisms:

1. deposition of insoluble $A\beta_{42}$ in the SP of the brain, which might be in part the result of disturbance of the clearance of $A\beta_{42}$
2. decrease of production of $A\beta_{42}$ by less (active) neurons, inevitably a result of neurodegeneration
3. altered binding to $A\beta_{42}$-specific proteins (e.g. Apo E), resulting in masking of the epitope, to which the antibodies of the assays are directed.

The decrease of CSF $A\beta_{42}$ concentration in AD is about 50% of that recorded in controls.[17] The most commonly used assay is the commercial ELISA of Innogenetics (Table 2.1). The median values of $A\beta_{42}$, as measured in two large case-control studies, are:

- AD = 487 (394–622) pg/ml, controls = 849 (682–1063) pg/ml;[18]
- AD = 394 (326–504) pg/ml, controls = 1076 (941–1231) pg/ml.[19]

Table 2.1 Diagnostic accuracy of cerebrospinal fluid (CSF) Aβ$_{42}$ and tau combined in Alzheimer's disease (AD) vs controls

Study	Population[a]	Gold standard[b]	Criteria[c]	Result	Cut off	Method
Galasko et al, 1998[22]	82 probable AD 60 controls	Clinical diagnosis (1A)	NINCDS–ADRDA	Sensitivity 77% Specificity 93%	Aβ$_{42}$: 1032 pg/ml Tau: 503 pg/ml	Aβ$_{42}$ and tau: in-house methods Multicenter study
Kanai et al, 1998[34]	93 probable AD 41 controls	Clinical diagnosis (1A)	NINCDS–ADRDA	Sensitivity 40% Specificity 90%	Aβ$_{42}$: 256 fmol/ml Tau: 474 pg/ml	Aβ$_{42}$: in-house method Tau: Innogenetics
Hulstaert et al, 1999[18]	150 probable AD 100 controls = 42 HC + 58 OND	Clinical diagnosis (1A)	NINCDS–ADRDA	Sensitivity 85% Specificity 86%	Aβ$_{42}$: 643 pg/ml Tau: 252 pg/ml	Aβ$_{42}$ and tau: Innogenetics Multicenter study
Tapiola et al, 2000[23]	80 probable AD 41 definite AD 39 OND	Clinical (1A) and neuropathologic diagnosis (1A)	NINCDS–ADRDA CERAD	Sensitivity 46–53%[d] Specificity 95%	Aβ$_{42}$: 340 pg/ml Tau: 380 pg/mlL	Aβ$_{42}$: in-house method Tau: Innogenetics
Andreasen et al, 2001[35]	105 probable AD 100 controls of Hulstaert et al.[18]	Clinical diagnosis (1A)	NINCDS–ADRDA	Sensitivity 94% Specificity 89%	Aβ$_{42}$: 643 pg/ml Tau: 252 pg/ml	Aβ$_{42}$ and tau: Innogenetics
Riemenschneider et al, 2002[19]	74 probable AD 40 controls	Clinical diagnosis (1A)	NINCDS–ADRDA	Sensitivity 92% Specificity 95%	Aβ$_{42}$: 738 pg/ml Tau: 255 pg/ml	Aβ$_{42}$ and tau: Innogenetics

[a] Probable AD = AD according to the clinical NINCDS–ADRDA criteria; definite AD = AD confirmed at neuropathologic examination; OND = other neurologic diseases.
[b] 1A = clinical diagnosis is gold standard, prospective collected materials, including groups of patients and controls with a minimum of 30 individuals; 1A = neuropathologic diagnose is gold standard, rest conform to class 1A.
[c] NINCDS–ADRDA = National Institute of Neurological and Communicative Diseases and Stroke/Alzheimer's Disease and Related Disorders Association.
[d] Definite and probable AD vs OND.

Table 2.1 Continued

Study	Population[a]	Gold standard[b]	Criteria[c]	Result	Cut off	Method
Kapaki et al, 2003[24]	49 probable AD 49 controls	Clinical diagnosis (1A) 3 year follow-up	NINCDS–ADRDA	Sensitivity 96% Specificity 86%	$A\beta_{42}$: 490 pg/ml Tau: 317 pg/ml	$A\beta_{42}$ and tau: Innogenetics
Sunderland et al, 2003[6]	131 probable AD 72 controls	Clinical diagnosis (1A)	DSM-IV NINCDS–ADRDA	Sensitivity 92% Specificity 89%	$A\beta_{42}$: 444 pg/ml Tau: 195 pg/ml	$A\beta_{42}$: in-house method Tau: Innogenetics

[a] Probable AD = AD according to the clinical NINCDS–ADRDA criteria; definite AD = AD confirmed at neuropathologic examination; OND = other neurologic diseases.
[b] 1A = clinical diagnosis is gold standard, prospective collected materials, including groups of patients and controls with a minimum of 30 individuals; 1A = neuropathologic diagnose is gold standard, rest conform to class 1A.
[c] NINCDS–ADRDA = National Institute of Neurological and Communicative Diseases and Stroke/Alzheimer's Disease and Related Disorders Association.
[d] Definite and probable AD vs OND.

Reference value for CSF $A\beta_{42}$ obtained from a control population is set above 500 pg/ml.[20] Sensitivity ranged from 69–100%, whereas specificity ranged from 56–85% in a subset of studies.[19,21–25] Considerable variability in absolute levels of $A\beta_{42}$ exists among centers, even when using the same commercial assay. Cross-sectional studies show little evidence of a relationship between CSF $A\beta_{42}$ and age, except for one study showing a U-shaped natural course in normal aging, with an increase of CSF $A\beta_{42}$ until 29 and over 60 years old.[26] No[18,23] or only a weak[22] cross-sectional relationship has been found between CSF $A\beta_{42}$ and disease duration or Mini-Mental State Examination (MMSE). Only one study investigated and found an association between the number of SPs and the CSF $A\beta_{42}$ concentration.[27]

Tau

Many studies have demonstrated that tau is increased in CSF of AD patients; concentrations are about three times higher in AD than in non-demented controls. However, there is a large variation in the range of CSF tau concentration in AD. Median and mean concentrations of CSF are 425 (274–713) pg/ml and 587 (365) pg/mL in AD, and 195 (121–294) pg/mL and 224 (156) pg/ml in controls.[6,18] The increase of tau in CSF is supposed to be the result of release from dying neurons containing a large number of NFTs. One study demonstrated that CSF tau concentration was related to the number of NFTs in the brain.[28]

Again, the most commonly used assay for tau is the ELISA from Innogenetics (Table 2.1). Mean sensitivity ranged from 55 to 81% at a mean specificity value of 90% comparing AD with controls.[17] Important is that CSF tau increases with age,[19,29] which stresses the need to compare only groups from the same age category.[30] Furthermore, CSF tau tends to be increased in several other neurologic disorders, such as acute stroke[31] and trauma,[32] indicating that the marker is not very specific. Reference values for tau in healthy individuals are defined as <300 pg/ml (21–50 years old); <450 pg/ml (51–70 years old); and <500 pg/ml (71–93 years old).[19] No correlation was found between CSF tau and MMSE or disease duration.

Combination of CSF $A\beta_{42}$ and tau

Diagnostic accuracy, especially the specificity, increases when using the combination of CSF $A\beta_{42}$ and tau comparing AD with controls, including patients with depression or memory problems due to alcohol abuse.[17] In Table 2.1 an overview is given of class IA and 1A case-control studies, with neuropathologic (IA) or clinical diagnosis (1A) as gold standard, and patient and control groups included with a minimum of 30 individuals.[33]

Isoprostanes

Oxidative stress is thought to play an important role in the cascade, resulting in cell death in AD.[36] A few studies have demonstrated that isoprostanes are increased in CSF of AD patients, even at an early stage of disease.[37,38] Further studies are needed on how these proteins can be used in the diagnostic work up for AD, especially to clarify the specificity of these markers.

CEREBROSPINAL FLUID MARKERS IN ALZHEIMER'S DISEASE VS OTHER DEMENTIAS

Combination of CSF $A\beta_{42}$ and tau

How good is the diagnostic accuracy when using the combination of $A\beta_{42}$ and tau in AD compared with other types of dementias? Although this topic is much more relevant for clinical practice, only a few studies investigated these two markers in large groups of patients. Most studies found a lower specificity as compared to the studies mentioned in Table 2.1. There is substantial overlap in CSF $A\beta_{42}$ and tau concentrations between different types of dementias. A decreased concentration of CSF $A\beta_{42}$ can be found in DLB, FTD, and VAD.[18,20,30,39] A high CSF tau is also not specific for AD: CSF tau is found to be increased in a subset of FTD and VAD patients.[18,30] In most cases of DLB, CSF tau concentration is normal.[39] In CJD, CSF $A\beta_{42}$ is decreased and CSF tau is found to be very high, even higher than in AD.[40] The specificity of the combined CSF $A\beta_{42}$/tau analysis varies from 85%, comparing AD with FTD, to 67%, in AD vs DLB, and 48%, in AD vs VAD (Table 2.2).

Phosphorylated tau

Several investigators have developed assays to detect phosphorylated tau (Ptau) in CSF. As NFTs have an abundance of abnormally phosphorylated tau, it is to be expected that Ptau is increased in CSF from AD patients. Several immunoassays have been developed that are specific for the phosphorylated epitopes threonine 181 (Ptau-181),[41] serine 199 (Ptau-199),[42] and threonine 231 (Ptau-231).[43] Good results have been obtained comparing AD with other types of dementia; in the majority of patients, Ptau is found to be normal in DLB,[44] VAD,[45] FTD,[30] and CJD.[46] One study demonstrated an increase in diagnostic accuracy of Ptau-231 and Ptau-181 compared to Ptau-199 in differentiating AD from other types of dementia.[47] The same authors found a decline of CSF Ptau-231 during the course of AD in 17 patients.[48] These data need to be confirmed in another independent study, preferably with postmortem confirmation of diagnoses. A greater diagnostic accuracy of Ptau compared with total tau is obtained in most studies.[30,49] In one study it has been shown that the combination of CSF $A\beta_{42}$ with Ptau-181 differentiated best early onset AD (EAD) from FTD with a high specificity (93%) and a low negative predictive

Table 2.2   Diagnostic accuracy of cerebrospinal fluid (CSF) and tau combined in Alzheimer's disease (AD) vs other types of dementia

Study	Population[a]	Gold standard[b]	Criteria[c]	Result	Cut off
Galasko et al, 1998[22]	82 probable AD 74 NAD	Clinical diagnosis (1A)	NINCDS–ADRDA	Sensitivity 77% Specificity 65%	$A\beta_{42}$: 1032 pg/ml Tau: 503 pg/ml
Hulstaert et al, 1999[18]	150 probable AD 79 NAD	Clinical diagnosis (1A)	NINCDS–ADRDA	Sensitivity 85% Specificity 58%	$A\beta_{42}$: 643 pg/ml Tau: 252 pg/ml
Tapiola, 2000[23]	80 probable AD 41 definite AD 27 NAD	Clinical (1A) and neuropathological diagnosis (1A)	NINCDS–ADRDA CERAD	Sensitivity 50% Specificity 85%	$A\beta_{42}$: 340 pg/ml Tau: 380 pg/ml
Andreasen et al, 2001[35]	105 probable AD 23 VAD 9 DLB	Clinical diagnosis (1A)	NINCDS–ADRDA VAD: NINDS–AIREN DLB: McKeith	Sensitivity 94% Specificity VAD 48% Specificity DLB 67%	$A\beta_{42}$: 643 pg/ml Tau: 252 pg/ml
Riemenschneider et al, 2002[19]	74 probable AD 34 FTLD	Clinical diagnosis (1A)	NINCDS–ADRDA FTLD: Neary	Sensitivity 85% Specificity 85%	$A\beta_{42}$: 528 pg/ml Tau: 432 pg/ml
Kapaki et al, 2003[24]	49 probable AD 15 NAD 6 VAD	Clinical diagnosis (1A)	NINCDS–ADRDA VAD: NINDS–AIREN AD vs NAD/VAD:	AD vs NAD: Sensitivity: 71–90% Specificity: 83–100%	$A\beta_{42}$: 435 pg/ml Tau: 437 pg/ml
Schoonenboom et al, 2004[30]	47 probable EAD 28 FTLD	Clinical diagnosis (1A)	NINCDS–ADRDA FTLD: Neary	Sensitivity 72% Specificity 89%	$A\beta_{42}$: 413 pg/ml Tau: 377 pg/ml

[a] Probable AD = AD according to the clinical NINCDS–ADRDA criteria; definite AD = AD confirmed at neuropathologic examination; EAD = early-onset AD, disease starting before 65 years old; VAD = vascular dementia; DLB = diffuse Lewy body disease; FTLD = frontotemporal lobar degeneration; NAD = non-Alzheimer dementia.
[b] 1A = clinical diagnosis is gold standard, prospective collected materials, including groups of patients and controls with a minimum of 30 individuals; 1A = neuropathologic diagnosis is gold standard, rest conform to class 1A.
[c] NINCDS–ADRDA = National Institute of Neurological and Communicative Diseases and Stroke/Alzheimer's Disease and Related Disorders Association. CERAD = Consortium to Establish a Register for Alzheimer's Disease. AIREN = Association Internationale pour la Recherche et l'Enseignement en Neurosciences.

value (negative likelihood ratio=0.03).[30] As there still exists overlap between the different types of dementia, either clinically or biochemically, a combination of the three markers seems best for routine clinical practice, with at least two of the three biomarkers positive as indicator for AD.[50]

14-3-3 protein

The 14-3-3 protein gives, like tau, a reflection of (fast progressive) neuron loss. It can be detected in CSF by the semiquantitative Western blot analysis. When used in the proper context, with a high clinical suspicion and in combination with electroencephalography (EEG), MRI scan, and routine CSF analysis, the measurement of 14-3-3 protein in CSF supports the diagnosis of CJD with high diagnostic accuracy.[51] False-positive results can be obtained in acute stroke, brain tumor, encephalitis, or even (fast progressive) AD. Sensitivity and specificity values of CSF 14-3-3 and tau have been reported to be the same in one study (cut-off level for tau=1300 pg/ml).[52] Recently, it has been shown that the combination of 14-3-3 protein and $A\beta_{42}$ gives the highest diagnostic accuracy for CJD (sensitivity 100%, specificity 98%, positive predictive value 93%, negative predictive value 100%).[40]

GOLD STANDARD

The majority of the above-mentioned studies have been obtained in groups of patients where the diagnosis has been obtained clinically. The accuracy of the clinical diagnosis in specialized settings is estimated at around 85%.[53] By use of clinical criteria, there is risk of circular reasoning: i.e. the diagnostic performance of CSF markers cannot be higher than the accuracy of the clinical criteria.[17] The NINCDS/ADRDA (National Institute of Neurological and Communicative Diseases and Stroke/Alzheimer's Disease and Related Disorders Association) criteria for AD have a high sensitivity but a moderately high specificity. Illustrative is the specificity of only 23% of the NINCDS/ADRDA criteria for the differentiation of AD from FTD in one retrospective neuropathologic study.[54] Furthermore, 40–80% of the clinically diagnosed VAD patients have concomitant AD pathology.[55] Only two studies were published in which (in part) the neuropathologic diagnosis was used as gold standard.[23,56] For the differentiation of AD from controls, similar sensitivity and specificity were obtained for CSF tau and $A\beta_{42}$ as compared to clinical studies (Table 2.1).[23] However, the specificity of FTD and DLB compared with AD was not optimal, 69%.[56]

Most published studies were performed in specialized tertiary referral settings with selected patient groups. Only a few studies were carried out with consecutively recruited patients from a memory clinic; sensitivity was high, but specificity was lower in this setting with 'unselected' patients.[35,57] More studies are needed in large primary and secondary referral centers to obtain an insight into how to use CSF $A\beta_{42}$, tau, and Ptau in an elderly population in clinical practice. Population-based studies are under way to establish CSF markers as potential biomarkers for routine diagnostic use

MILD COGNITIVE IMPAIRMENT

Mild cognitive impairment (MCI) is considered to be a transitional state between normal aging and dementia. Around 10–15% of MCI patients progress to Alzheimer-type dementia each year.[58] Several studies have shown that a subgroup of MCI patients has low CSF $A\beta_{42}$ levels and/or high CSF tau levels at baseline that are indicative for AD.[17] Furthermore, there is evidence that these markers can be used as predictors for the conversion of MCI to AD.[50,59] It is not clear yet which marker is changed first in the disease process, as contradictory findings are reported by various studies describing either an increased CSF tau[50,60] or a decreased CSF $A\beta_{42}$ at baseline.[61,62] In two independent studies a relationship between CSF tau with memory impairment was found, whereas this was not the case for CSF $A\beta_{42}$.[63,64] Good results have been obtained for CSF Ptau as an indicator of AD-related changes in the MCI stage.[4,59,65] In one study it has been demonstrated that high CSF levels of Ptau at baseline, but not CSF tau levels, correlated with cognitive decline and conversion of MCI to AD.[66] A very recent study, following 78 MCI patients, shows the best prediction for the development of AD using the combination of CSF $A\beta_{42}$ with Ptau.[67] Most of the studies mentioned have been conducted retrospectively in research settings, and limited data are available about the frequency of a biomarker profile typical for AD in a prospective setting that reflects clinical practice. But, overall, the use of biomarkers in combination with other diagnostic tools is very promising in recognizing MCI patients who will develop AD in the future.

NEUROIMAGING AND CEREBROSPINAL FLUID BIOMARKER STUDIES

Cross-sectional studies

Hippocampal size reduction, atrophy of the medial temporal lobe (MTL), and the entorhinal cortex (EC) are sensitive markers for AD. Moreover, atrophy of the hippocampus is found to be a good predictor in MCI for the development of AD. However, these markers are not disease-specific and cannot be used as primary evidence for AD.[4] By combining CSF and MRI markers, one could get a better diagnostic accuracy. In addition, by investigating the relationship between the two markers a better understanding of the agreement between the two disease markers could be obtained: do they reflect the same pathologic substrate at the same time? Only a few studies have investigated the cross-sectional relationship between CSF biomarkers and atrophy on MRI in small groups of patients. One study showed a correlation between CSF $A\beta_{42}$ and the volume of the temporal lobes.[68] We were unable to find a relationship between atrophy of the MTL and CSF $A\beta_{42}$, tau, and Ptau in 62 mild–moderate AD patients and 32 controls when considered as separate groups.[69] Moreover, both disease markers contributed independently to the diagnosis of AD. In MCI patients, we found a relationship between CSF $A\beta_{42}$ and atrophy of the MTL, whereas CSF tau did not relate to MTA.[63] These data corresponded to a larger study reporting lower baseline CSF $A\beta_{42}$ levels with lower brain volume and larger ventricular volume in the spectrum of normal aging, MCI, and AD.[70] In contrast, higher CSF tau and Ptau were found with an increase in ventricular widening during follow-up. In this light, CSF $A\beta_{42}$ can be more considered as a *stage* marker, indicating the presence of disease at a certain time, whereas CSF tau is more a *state* marker, indicating the intensity of the neuronal damage and degeneration.[17,70] However, these data give only information about one time point in the disease, and until now it has not been possible to show progressive changes in CSF $A\beta_{42}$ or Ptau concentrations, except for one study.[71] On the other hand, atrophy rates on MRI are good indicators of disease progression in MCI and AD. The question is therefore: can both disease markers be used as markers of progression?

Longitudinal studies

The few studies investigating the change in CSF biomarkers were carried out on AD patients. Little is known about the change of CSF $A\beta_{42}$, tau, and Ptau in MCI, whereas one would expect that in this early stage of disease the biomarkers would be more prone to change than in later stages. One study investigated whether there was a longitudinal relationship between the change in biomarkers with the change in hippocampal volume on MRI in a small group of aged individuals with and without memory problems.[4] In a two time-point longitudinal design, the MCI group, $n = 8$, showed an inverse relationship between hippocampal volume reductions and elevations in CSF Ptau, whereas CSF $A\beta_{42}$ levels showed a positive relationship with hippocampal volume reductions. However, there are several limitations of this study:

- a very small group was investigated
- it is not known whether these MCI patients will develop AD
- and the change in biomarkers could also be due to the intra-assay variability, as very small changes are detected.

Indeed, the authors did not find a significant change in CSF $A\beta_{42}$, and Ptau concentrations between two time points if they corrected for dilution of tau due to ventricular enlargement; this 'Ptau-231 load' was increased in MCI at follow-up.[65] These findings need to be replicated in larger groups of patients; in addition, further studies are warranted for a better understanding of the CSF flow and clearance dynamics of biomarkers.

ADDED VALUE OF CEREBROSPINAL FLUID MARKERS OVER OTHER DIAGNOSTIC TOOLS

In a recent review the position of CSF markers in the clinical assessment of patients with MCI and early AD has been discussed.[17] The authors suggest that only after intensive screening of the patients by history, neurologic examination, routine laboratory tests (blood and CSF), and neuroimaging (computed tomography (CT), MRI, or single-photon emission computed tomography (SPECT)) is there a place for CSF markers for the (early) diagnosis of AD. The clinical diagnosis of AD should be based on the cumulative information of all the different diagnostic tools, as in other areas of medicine. For the differential diagnosis of AD, we state that the biomarkers are especially important for the early-onset dementias, as there is clinical and radiologic overlap, especially between EAD and FTD. In the older age group, the prevalence of AD is much higher, and the usefulness of biomarkers to distinguish AD from other types of dementia becomes less relevant. However, since the currently available medications to enhance cognition are approved for mild to moderate AD, every hint to the correct diagnosis should be taken into account irrespective of age. The added value of CSF markers over other diagnostic tools has not yet been investigated systematically, and is an aim for future studies.

LIMITATIONS OF RESEARCH ON CEREBROSPINAL FLUID MARKERS

For the differentiation of AD from normal aging, depression, or other types of dementia, overlap is seen in CSF $A\beta_{42}$, tau, and Ptau concentrations between the groups. One explanation is that the control or demented groups could have neuropathologic findings indicative for AD, resulting in an AD biomarker profile. It is also not yet clear whether the decrease of CSF $A\beta_{42}$ and the increase of (P)tau actually reflect the plaques and tangles in AD. Other explanations are the use of different processing and storage conditions of CSF between different centers,[72] the use of different reagent antibodies, differences in the definition of cut-off values, and intra- and inter-assay variability of the assays used.[17] Standardization of the (pre-) analytical methods will increase the reliability of the results and improve collaboration with other neurologic/biochemical research centers or memory clinics. Although it is not difficult to obtain CSF by lumbar puncture, this method is considered to be somewhat invasive for an outpatient clinic, especially in the USA. Therefore, a sensitive serum or plasma marker for AD would be very valuable for use in clinical practice.

CONCLUSION

For the differentiation of AD from normal aging, depression, or alcoholic dementia, the combination of CSF $A\beta_{42}$ with tau gives a high sensitivity and specificity of ≥85%, with minimal overlap in individual cases. In the pre-clinical (MCI) stage of disease, CSF $A\beta_{42}$, tau, and Ptau could be used as predictors for the development of AD. For the differentiation of AD from other types of dementia, the combination of CSF $A\beta_{42}$, tau, and Ptau gives a good sensitivity and a reasonable specificity, especially for the differentiation of AD from FTD and less for AD vs DLB or VAD. For clinical practice, a high positive predictive value and a low negative predictive value are important. With at least two markers positive, the diagnosis of AD is very likely, while two markers negative could practically rule out diagnosis of AD. The CSF biomarkers must only be used in combination with other diagnostic tools, including clinical history and examination, imaging, and neuropsychologic work-up.

Guidelines for the use of CSF $A\beta_{42}$, tau and Ptau in clinical practice

1. When there is doubt about the diagnosis AD, with non-conclusive MRI or neuropsychological findings.
2. In patients with early-onset dementias (disease onset before 65 years old), as the differential diagnosis here is wider and more complicated; in particular, the differentiation of EAD from FTD is relevant.
3. In patients suspected for CJD, in combination with CSF 14-3-3 protein, MRI scan, and EEG.

Topics for future research

*   Investigate the additional value of the biomarkers CSF $A\beta_{42}$, tau, and Ptau to other diagnostic methods, i.e. MRI parameters and/or neuropsychologic examinations.
*   Investigate the diagnostic value of the biomarkers in primary and secondary referral settings, preferably with neuropathologic or prolonged clinical follow-up.
*   Investigate which markers could be used for tracking the progression of the disease, especially in the MCI stage of disease. Promising markers are C- and N-terminally truncated $A\beta$ peptides, oxidative stress markers or inflammatory markers.
*   Develop new tests for a sensitive marker that can be determined in blood or urine.
*   Standardize (pre-analytical) laboratory methods between research centers.

REFERENCES

1. Stevens T, Livingston G, Kitchen G, et al. Islington study of dementia subtypes in the community. Br J Psychiatry 2002;180:270–276.

2. Hebert LE, Scherr PA, Bienias JL, Bennett DA, Evans DA. Alzheimer disease in the US population: prevalence estimates using the 2000 census. Arch Neurol 2003;60: 1119–1122.

3. McKhann G, Drachman D, Folstein M, et al. Clinical diagnosis of Alzheimer's disease: report of the NINCDS-ADRDA Work Group under the auspices of Department of Health and Human Services Task Force on Alzheimer's Disease. Neurology 1984;34:939–944.

4. de Leon MJ, De Santi S, Zinkowski R, et al. MRI and CSF studies in the early diagnosis of Alzheimer's disease. J Int Med 2004;256:205–223.

5. Citron M. Strategies for disease modification in Alzheimer's disease. Nat Rev Neurosci 2004;5:677–685.

6. Sunderland T, Linker G, Mirza N, et al. Decreased beta-amyloid1-42 and increased tau levels in cerebrospinal fluid of patients with Alzheimer disease. JAMA 2003;289:2094–2103.

7. Consensus report of the Working Group on: "Molecular and Biochemical Markers of Alzheimer's Disease". The Ronald and Nancy Reagan Research Institute of the Alzheimer's Association and the National Institute on Aging Working Group. Neurobiol Aging 1998; 19:109–116.

8. Braak H, Braak E. Evolution of neuronal changes in the course of Alzheimer's disease. J Neural Transm Suppl 1998;53:127–140.

9. Braak H, Braak E. Evolution of the neuropathology of Alzheimer's disease. Acta Neurol Scand Suppl 1996;165:3–12.

10. Arriagada PV, Marzloff K, Hyman BT. Distribution of Alzheimer-type pathologic changes in nondemented elderly individuals matches the pattern in Alzheimer's disease. Neurology 1992;42(9):1681–1688.

11. McKhann GM, Albert MS, Grossman M, et al. Work Group on Frontotemporal Dementia and Pick's Disease. Clinical and pathological diagnosis of frontotemporal dementia: report of the Work Group on Frontotemporal Dementia and Pick's Disease. Arch Neurol 2001;58: 1803–1809.

12. Budka H, Aguzzi A, Brown P, et al. Neuropathological diagnostic criteria for Creutzfeldt–Jakob disease (CJD) and other human spongiform encephalopathies (prion diseases). Brain Pathol 1995;5:459–466.

13. McKeith IG, Galasko D, Kosaka K, et al. Consensus guidelines for the clinical and pathologic diagnosis of dementia with Lewy bodies (DLB): report of the consortium on DLB international workshop. Neurology 1996;47:1113–1124.

14. Vinters HV, Ellis WG, Zarow C, et al. Neuropathologic substrates of ischemic vascular dementia. J Neuropathol Exp Neurol 2000;59: 931–945.

15. Cummings JL. Towards a molecular neuropsychiatry of neurodegenerative diseases. Ann Neurol 2003; 54:147–154.

16. Englund E. Neuropathology of white matter changes in Alzheimer's disease and vascular dementia. Dement Geriatr Cogn Disord 1998;9(Suppl 1):6–12.

17. Blennow K, Hampel H. CSF markers for incipient Alzheimer's disease. Lancet Neurol 2003;2:605–613.

18. Hulstaert F, Blennow K, Ivanoiu A, et al. Improved discrimination of AD

patients using beta-amyloid(1-42) and tau levels in CSF. Neurology 1999;52:1555–1562.

19. Riemenschneider M, Wagenpfeil S, Diehl J, et al. Tau and Abeta42 protein in CSF of patients with frontotemporal degeneration. Neurology 2002;58:1622–1628.

20. Sjogren M, Vanderstichele H, Agren H, et al. Tau and Abeta42 in cerebrospinal fluid from healthy adults 21–93 years of age: establishment of reference values. Clin Chem 2001;47:1776–1781.

21. Motter R, Vigo-Pelfrey C, Kholodenko D, et al. Reduction of beta-amyloid peptide42 in the cerebrospinal fluid of patients with Alzheimer's disease. Ann Neurol 1995;38:643–648.

22. Galasko D, Chang L, Motter R, et al. High cerebrospinal fluid tau and low amyloid beta42 levels in the clinical diagnosis of Alzheimer disease and relation to apolipoprotein E genotype. Arch Neurol 1998; 55:937–945.

23. Tapiola T, Pirttila T, Mehta PD, et al. Relationship between Apo E genotype and CSF beta-amyloid (1-42) and tau in patients with probable and definite Alzheimer's disease. Neurobiol Aging 2000;21:735–740.

24. Kapaki E, Paraskevas GP, Zalonis I, Zournas C. CSF tau protein and beta-amyloid (1-42) in Alzheimer's disease diagnosis: discrimination from normal ageing and other dementias in the Greek population. Eur J Neurol 2003;10:119–128.

25. Ganzer S, Arlt S, Schroder V, et al. CSF-tau, CSF-Aβ1-42, ApoE-genotype and clinical parameters in the diagnosis of Alzheimer's disease: combination of CSF-tau and MMSE yields highest sensitivity and specificity. J Neural Transm 2003;110: 1149–1160.

26. Shoji M, Kanai M, Matsubara E, et al. The levels of cerebrospinal fluid Abeta40 and Abeta42(43) are regulated age-dependently. Neurobiol Aging 2001;22:209–221.

27. Strozyk D, Blennow K, White LR, Launer LJ. CSF Abeta 42 levels correlate with amyloid-neuropathology in a population-based autopsy study. Neurology 2003;60:652–656.

28. Tapiola T, Overmyer M, Lehtovirta M, et al. The level of cerebrospinal fluid tau correlates with neurofibrillary tangles in Alzheimer's disease. Neuroreport 1997 8:3961–3963.

29. Buerger nee Buch K, Padberg F, Nolde T, et al. Cerebrospinal fluid tau protein shows a better discrimination in young old (<70 years) than in old old patients with Alzheimer's disease compared with controls. Neurosci Lett 1999;277:21–24.

30. Schoonenboom NS, Pijnenburg YA, Mulder C, et al. Amyloid beta (1-42) and phosphorylated tau in CSF as markers for early-onset Alzheimer disease. Neurology 2004;62: 1580–1584.

31. Hesse C, Rosengren L, Vanmechelen E, et al. Cerebrospinal fluid markers for Alzheimer's disease evaluated after acute ischemic stroke. J Alzheimers Dis 2000;2:199–206.

32. Franz G, Beer R, Kampfl A, et al. Amyloid beta 1-42 and tau in cerebrospinal fluid after severe traumatic brain injury. Neurology 2003; 60:1457–1461.

33. Qizilbash N, ed. Evidence-based Dementia Practice. Oxford: Blackwell Science, 2002.

34. Kanai M, Matsubara E, Isoe K, et al. Longitudinal study of cerebrospinal fluid levels of tau, A beta1-40, and A beta1-42(43) in Alzheimer's disease: a study in Japan. Ann Neurol 1998;44:17–26

35. Andreasen N, Minthon L, Davidsson P, et al. Evaluation of CSF-tau and CSF-Abeta42 as diagnostic markers for Alzheimer disease in clinical practice. Arch Neurol 2001;58: 373–379.

36. Cutler RG, Kelly J, Storie K, et al. Involvement of oxidative stress-induced abnormalities in ceramide and cholesterol metabolism in brain

aging and Alzheimer's disease. Proc Natl Acad Sci USA 2004;101:2070–2075.

37. Montine KS, Quinn JF, Zhang J, et al. Isoprostanes and related products of lipid peroxidation in neurodegenerative diseases. Chem Phys Lipids 2004;128:117–124.

38. Pratico D, Clark CM, Lee VM, et al. Increased 8,12-iso-iPF2alpha-VI in Alzheimer's disease: correlation of a noninvasive index of lipid peroxidation with disease severity. Ann Neurol 2000;48:809–812.

39. Kanemaru K, Kameda N, Yamanouchi H. Decreased CSF amyloid beta42 and normal tau levels in dementia with Lewy bodies. Neurology 2000;54:1875–1876.

40. Van Everbroeck B, Quoilin S, Boons J, Martin JJ, Cras P. A prospective study of CSF markers in 250 patients with possible Creutzfeldt–Jakob disease. J Neurol Neurosurg Psychiatry 2003;74:1210–1214.

41. Vanmechelen E, Vanderstichele H, Davidsson P, et al. Quantification of tau phosphorylated at threonine 181 in human cerebrospinal fluid: a sandwich ELISA with a synthetic phosphopeptide for standardization. Neurosci Lett 2000;285:49–52.

42. Itoh N, Arai H, Urakami K, et al. Large-scale, multicenter study of cerebrospinal fluid tau protein phosphorylated at serine 199 for the antemortem diagnosis of Alzheimer's disease. Ann Neurol 2001;50:150–156.

43. Kohnken R, Buerger K, Zinkowski R, et al. Detection of tau phosphorylated at threonine 231 in cerebrospinal fluid of Alzheimer's disease patients. Neurosci Lett 2000;287:187–190.

44. Parnetti L, Lanari A, Amici S, et al. CSF phosphorylated tau is a possible marker for discriminating Alzheimer's disease from dementia with Lewy bodies. Phospho-Tau International Study Group. Neurol Sci 2001;22:77–78.

45. Nagga K, Gottfries J, Blennow K, Marcusson J. Cerebrospinal fluid phospho-tau, total tau and beta-amyloid(1-42) in the differentiation between Alzheimer's disease and vascular dementia. Dement Geriatr Cogn Disord 2002;14:183–190.

46. Riemenschneider M, Wagenpfeil S, Vanderstichele H, et al. Phospho-tau/total tau ratio in cerebrospinal fluid discriminates Creutzfeldt–Jakob disease from other dementias. Mol Psychiatry 2003;8:343–347.

47. Hampel H, Buerger K, Zinkowski R, et al. Measurement of phosphorylated tau epitopes in the differential diagnosis of Alzheimer disease: a comparative cerebrospinal fluid study. Arch Gen Psychiatry 2004;61:95–102.

48. Hampel H, Buerger K, Kohnken R, et al. Tracking of Alzheimer's disease progression with cerebrospinal fluid tau protein phosphorylated at threonine 231. Ann Neurol 2001;49:545–546.

49. Buerger K, Zinkowski R, Teipel SJ, et al. Differential diagnosis of Alzheimer disease with cerebrospinal fluid levels of tau protein phosphorylated at threonine 231. Arch Neurol 2002;59:1267–1272.

50. Zetterberg H, Wahlund LO, Blennow K. Cerebrospinal fluid markers for prediction of Alzheimer's disease. Neurosci Lett 2003;352:67–69.

51. Lemstra AW, van Meegen M, Baas F, van Gool WA. Clinical algorithm for cerebrospinal fluid test of 14-3-3 protein in diagnosis of Creutzfeldt–Jakob disease. Ned Tijdschr Geneeskd 2001;145:1467–1471.

52. Otto M, Wiltfang J, Cepek L, et al. Tau protein and 14-3-3 protein in the differential diagnosis of Creutzfeldt–Jakob disease. Neurology 2002;58:192–197.

53. Galasko D, Hansen LA, Katzmann R, et al. Clinical-neuropathological correlations in Alzheimer's disease and

related dementias. Arch Neurol 1994;51:888–895.

54. Varma AR, Snowden JS, Lloyd JJ, et al. Evaluation of the NINCDS–ADRDA criteria in the differentiation of Alzheimer's disease and frontotemporal dementia. J Neurol Neurosurg Psychiatry 1999; 66:184–188.

55. Jellinger KA. Diagnostic accuracy of Alzheimer's disease: a clinicopathological study. Acta Neuropath 1996;91:219–220.

56. Clark CM, Xie S, Chittams J, et al. Cerebrospinal fluid tau and beta-amyloid: how well do these biomarkers reflect autopsy-confirmed dementia diagnoses? Arch Neurol 2003;60:1696–1702.

57. Parnetti L, Lanari A, Saggese E, Spaccatini C, Gallai V. Cerebrospinal fluid biochemical markers in early detection and in differential diagnosis of dementia disorders in routine clinical practice. Neurol Sci 2003;24:199–200.

58. Petersen RC, Smith GE, Waring SC, et al. Mild cognitive impairment. Arch Neurol 1999;56:303–308.

59. Andreasen N, Vanmechelen E, Vanderstichele H, Davidsson P, Blennow K. Cerebrospinal fluid levels of total-tau, phospho-tau and A beta 42 predicts development of Alzheimer's disease in patients with mild cognitive impairment. Acta Neurol Scand Suppl 2003;179:47–51.

60. Maruyama M, Arai H, Sugita M, et al. Cerebrospinal fluid amyloid beta (1-42) in the mild cognitive impairment stage of Alzheimer's disease. Exp Neurol 2001;172;433–436.

61. Hampel H, Teipel SJ, Fuchsberger T, et al. Value of CSF beta-amyloid1-42 and tau as predictors of Alzheimer's disease in patients with mild cognitive impairment. Mol Psychiatry 2004;9:705–710.

62. Skoog I, Davidsson P, Aevarsson O, et al. Cerebrospinal fluid beta-amyloid 42 is reduced before the onset of sporadic dementia: a population-based study in 85-year-olds. Dement Geriatr Cogn Disord 2003;15: 169–176.

63. Schoonenboom SN, Visser PJ, Mulder C, et al. Biomarker profiles and their relation to clinical variables in mild cognitive impairment. Neurocase 2005;11:8–13.

64. Ivanoiu A, Sindic CJ. Cerebrospinal fluid TAU protein and amyloid beta42 in mild cognitive impairment: prediction of progression to Alzheimer's disease and correlation with the neuropsychological examination. Neurocase 2005;11:32–39.

65. de Leon MJ, Segal S, Tarshish CY, et al. Longitudinal cerebrospinal fluid tau load increases in mild cognitive impairment. Neurosci Lett 2002;333: 183–186.

66. Buerger K, Teipel SJ, Zinkowski R, et al. CSF tau protein phosphorylated at threonine 231 correlates with cognitive decline in MCI subjects. Neurology 2002;59:627–629.

67. Herukka SK, Hallikainen M, Soininen H, Pirttila T. CSF Abeta42 and tau or phosphorylated tau and prediction of progressive mild cognitive impairment. Neurology 2005;64: 1294–1297.

68. Schroder J, Pantel J, Ida N, et al. Cerebral changes and cerebrospinal fluid beta-amyloid in Alzheimer's disease: a study with quantitative magnetic resonance imaging. Mol Psychiatry 1997;2:505–507.

69. Schoonenboom NS, Barkhof F, Van der Flier WM, Blankenstein MA, Scheltens P. CSF markers and their relation to medial temporal lobe atrophy in Alzheimer's disease. Abstract AAN, Miami Beach, 2005.

70. Wahlund LO, Blennow K. Cerebrospinal fluid biomarkers for disease stage and intensity in cognitively impaired patients. Neurosci Lett 2003;339:99–102.

71. Tapiola T, Pirttila T, Mikkonen M, Three-year follow-up of cerebrospinal fluid tau, beta-amyloid 42 and 40 concentrations in Alzheimer's disease. Neurosci Lett 2000;280: 119–122.

72. Schoonenboom NS, Mulder C, Vanderstichele H, et al. Effects of processing and storage conditions on CSF amyloid beta (1-42) and tau concentrations: implications for use in clinical practice. Clin Chem 2005;51:189–195.

3

Executive control function in 'mild' cognitive impairment and Alzheimer's disease

Donald R Royall

INTRODUCTION

The term 'mild cognitive impairment' (MCI) has been applied to non-demented elderly persons with isolated cognitive and minimal functional impairment.[1] It is widely held that MCI progresses towards dementia, presumably that of Alzheimer's disease (AD).[2]

For the purposes of MCI case finding, cognitive 'impairment' is most often defined by a performance 1.0–1.5 standard deviations below an age-specific norm. When applied to memory test scores, this definition results in the selection of cases with an increased risk of dementia conversion. In an evidence-based review of MCI, the American Academy of Neurology cited six papers reporting conversion rates ranging from 6–25% per year.[2]

Although memory impairment has been the major focus of MCI research, it is increasingly clear that non-amnestic MCI syndromes also exist.[3] Whether non-amnestic MCI progresses to AD is debatable. AD pathology – i.e. neuro-fibrillary tangles (NFTs) and paired-helical filament tauopathy[*] – is hierarchically distributed in space, and presumably time.[4] The hippocampus is affected relatively early in this progression. This explains both the significance of isolated memory impairment as a harbinger of future AD, and the fact that memory impairment is almost universally present among cases with AD, as opposed to certain non-AD dementias. However, the hierarchical distribution of AD pathology also suggests that non-amnestic MCI is not likely to be AD related.

Impairment of executive control function (ECF) is likely to be common among persons diagnosed with MCI. First, ECF impairment is present both early in AD, but particularly in non-AD dementias. Secondly, it is increasingly clear that ECF impairment is common in medically ill and community-dwelling older persons at risk to be diagnosed with MCI.

---

[*]Senile plaque (SP) and β-amyloid are more randomly distributed and not always co-localized with NFT. However, regional NFT counts are more strongly correlated with AD's clinical features than are SP and fully mediate SP's unadjusted associations with cognition in multivariate models.

However, ECF, rather than memory loss, appears to a major predictor of functional outcomes. Thus, the issue of ECF impairment has implications for dementia case-finding that go well beyond 'MCI'. In contrast to memory or other non-executive cognitive impairments, the presence of ECF impairment suggests disability, and thus 'dementia' as well. The recognition of ECF impairment as being 'essential' to dementia would have far-ranging consequences for the epidemiology of that condition.

This chapter examines the issue of ECF impairments in both AD and MCI and considers the following questions:

- Is ECF impairment present in AD?
- Is ECF impairment reported in 'MCI'?
- Is ECF impairment likely to be present in 'amnestic' MCI?
- Can ECF impairment be observed in the absence of disability?
- Is isolated ECF impairment a true 'dementia'?

IS EXECUTIVE CONTROL FUNCTION IMPAIRMENT PRESENT IN ALZHEIMER'S DISEASE?

There is good reason to suspect that ECF impairment is present from the outset of *clinical* AD. First, frontal cortical AD pathology is more strongly related to cognitive impairment than are lesions in other regions of interest (ROIs). Plaques and tangles counted in the frontal cortex explain almost twice as much variance in cognition than do the same lesions in other ROIs.[5] Frontal lobe synaptic density is the strongest reported pathologic correlate of cognitive impairment in the AD literature.[6] In contrast, hippocampal AD pathology is relatively weakly associated with cognition, and may have no association with clinical dementia, independent of frontal lesions.[5]

A few multivariate models have been published that specifically associate regional AD pathology with clinical features of dementia. Geddes et al[7] factor-analyzed the regional distribution of NFTs. Two factors were identified. The first contained only mesiotemporal ROI, affected before Braak stage IV. This factor was significantly associated with memory impairment, but not dementia. In contrast, dementia was more closely associated with pathology in neocortical ROI, including the frontal cortex. Royall et al[8] modeled the individual contribution of regional tauopathy with clinical 'dementia', defined by a Clinical Dementia Rating (CDR) scale[9] score ≥ 1.0. The hippocampus was the only ROI whose pathology had no unadjusted association with dementia. 'Dementia' was most strongly associated with pathology in only four ROI, including the dorsolateral prefrontal cortex (Brodmann area (BA) 9/10), the angular gyrus (BA 39), the posterior cingulate (BA 23), and the superior temporal gyrus (BA 22). Each is retrogradely labeled by an excitotoxic lesion to the dorsolateral prefrontal cortex,[10] suggesting that they (and the anterior cingulate, not available to Royall et al[8]) comprise a single system focused on the executive control of complex behavior.[11] Diminished cerebral blood flow (rCBF), by functional magnetic resonance imaging (fMRI), in the same ROI, distinguishes AD, and apolipoprotein E (APOE) ε4 homozygotes, from non-demented elderly controls.[12]

Dementia can be diagnosed before the appearance of NFTs in neocortical ROIs.[13] However, this may require comorbid pathology.[11] In dementia cases, Braak stage is inversely related to the severity of comorbid ischemic cerebrovascular disease (ICVD)[14] and only a fraction of demented persons have *only* AD pathology at autopsy.[15] Moreover, the ischemic lesions with the strongest associations to cognition may be too small to image by computed tomography (CT) or MRI. Thus, 'mixed' cases may be misascribed to 'AD'.[16] However, since clinical dementia can also be specifically associated with 'strategic' infarcts involving the very same neocortical ROIs as AD,[17] and since neocortical function can be vicariously affected by subcortical frontal system lesions (i.e. through diaschisis)[18] it seems likely that clinical 'AD' is associated with frontal system dysfunction regardless of whether neocortical ROIs have been directly affected by AD pathology, or indirectly affected by comorbid ICVD.[19]

Nevertheless, there are surprisingly few data on ECF impairment in AD. Older studies either ignore this domain entirely, or use measures that have little sensitivity to ECF. Some more recent studies include executive measures. Lowenstein et al.[20] failed to find significant associations between some ECF measures – i.e. verbal fluency, digit-symbol substitution, or Weschler Adult Intelligence Scale (Revised) (WAIS-R) similarities – and the Direct Assessment of Functional Status (DAFS) in AD cases. Willis et al.[21] reported that ECF measures add variance to functional outcomes above that attributed to 'general' cognitive measures, but the additional variance explained was relatively small. Chen et al.[22] reported signifiant associations between Mattis Dementia Rating Scale (mDRS) 'initiation /perseveration' (I/P), mDRS 'conceptualization', and the number of categories achieved on the Wisconsin Card Sorting Test (WCST:CAT) and Blessed Dementia Scale: Activities subscale (BDS-A). Boyle et al.[23] report that the mDRS I/P explains 17% of variance in IADL (Instrumental Activities of Daily Living), and 9% of variance in ADL (Activities of Daily Living), independent of 'apathy' as measured by the Frontal System Behavior (FrSBe) scale.

In contrast, Marson et al.[24] report that mDRS I/P explained 36% of the variance in a 'rational reasons' standard of medical decision-making among AD patients. Similarly, the same group reported that verbal fluency explained 58% of variance in an 'Appreciating Consequences' standard.[25]

These studies suggest that although ECF impairment can be demonstrated in AD, its association with functional status varies widely with both the specific ECF measure employed and the functional outcome under consideration. IADL may be more strongly related to ECF than ADL, but ECF is most strongly related to 'higher' functional capacities, such as decision-making.

IS EXECUTIVE CONTROL FUNCTION IMPAIRMENT REPORTED IN MILD COGNITIVE IMPAIRMENT?

Very few studies have specifically addressed ECF impairment in the context of MCI. Nagahama et al.[26] factor-analyzed WCST performance in a small number of AD and MCI cases. Both groups were more executively impaired than normal controls, but they were not discriminable from each other on the basis of their perseverative errors. The MCI group actually made significantly more non-perseverative errors than the AD group. Similarly, Ready et al.[27] studied the rate of change in ECF-related behaviors (i.e. apathy, 'executive dysfunction', and disinhibition) in AD and MCI. Apathy and 'executive dysfunction' both increased over time, but MCI could not be distinguished from AD on the basis of these changes. Thus, it appears that ECF impairments comparable to AD can develop in the absence of a clinical diagnosis of 'dementia'.

To some extent, this is an artifact of dementia case definitions themselves. These emphasize the clinical detection of AD at the expense of non-AD conditions.[28] By definition, isolated ECF impairment cannot be classified as 'dementia' by either the DSM (Diagnostic and Statistical Manual)[29] or the NINCDS (National Institute of Neurological and Communicative Diseases and Stroke),[30] due to the absence of memory impairment. Conversely, clinical AD is unlikely to cause ECF impairment unless and until the hippocampus is affected at about Braak stage III.

This constraint forces researchers to place isolated ECF impairment into "non-demented" diagnostic categories (e.g. Age-Associated Cognitive Decline or Cognitive Impairment: No Dementia). A more subtle bias is the failure of clinicians to consider dementia when the clinical features of AD (i.e. aphasia, amnesia, and agnosia, which reflect a widespread cortical disease process) are not present. For example, Schillerstrom et al[31] tested ECF in N = 50 medical inpatients referred for psychiatric consultation (mean age = 44.9 ± 16.7 years). Although 62% were executively impaired (including 100% of cases diagnosed with dementia), only 22% were diagnosed by the psychiatrists as having cognitive impairment. In the absence of AD's clinical features, the consultants failed to recognize ECF's contribution to the other cases' behavioral changes.

Schillerstrom et al.[31] used the Executive Interview (EXIT25)[32] to identify patients with ECF impairment. The EXIT25's threshold for impairment (i.e. 15/50) is not age-adjusted. Instead, it was set to detect functional incapacity. The EXIT25 has previously been shown to be a significant independent predictor of IADL[33] and level of care[33,34] among elderly retirees. Dymek et al.[35] have reported that the EXIT25 independently accounted for 56% *of the variance* in the capacity of patients with Parkinson's disease to understand the circumstances and choices associated with their treatment, and 45% of the variance in a 'rational reasons' standard of the capacity to give informed consent. EXIT25 scores are also associated with medication adherence in medical patients.[36,37] Allen et al.[37] report that, at a cut-point of 15 /50, the EXIT25 perfectly distinguishes between elderly patients who can, and cannot, be taught to competently use inhalers.

However, the mean EXIT25 score for non-institutionalized, affluent, well-educated elderly retirees is about 12.5 /50.[33] Thus, although statistically 'normal' for their age, *38% will fail the EXIT25 at 15/50*, compared with 25% of community-dwelling young adults with schizophrenia,[38] 19.9% of cancer patients presenting for radiotherapy,[39] 42% of consecutively admitted medical inpatients,[40] and 59% of medical outpatients with type 2 diabetes mellitus.[41] Thus, ECF impairment sufficient to interfere with many aspects of healthcare delivery is likely to be quite common in medical settings. Moreover, in each of the studies cited above, Mini-Mental State Examination (MMSE) scores[42] *were within the normal range* (i.e. ≤24/30). In the absence of formal ECF testing, the lack of impairment in other domains can blind clinicians to the possibility of disabling ECF impairment.

IS EXECUTIVE CONTROL FUNCTION IMPAIRMENT LIKELY TO BE PRESENT IN 'AMNESTIC' MILD COGNITIVE IMPAIRMENT?

Some authors distinguish between 'amnestic' MCI, in which the cognitive impairments are limited to memory function, and more generalized 'mild' cognitive impairments. Nonetheless, it is likely that many 'amnestic' MCI cases actually do have both comorbid ECF impairments and disability. Depending on the measures employed, 25–35% of 'amnestic' MCI cases can be shown to have equally severe ECF impairment.[43] Such cases could arguably meet criteria for 'dementia' were either their disability or their ECF to be more rigorously assessed. For example, whereas the slope of change in the memory test scores of non-demented retirees is specifically associated with conversion to cortical-type dementias,[44] and is accelerated by the APOE ε4 allele,[45] simultaneous changes in ECF mediate memory's unadjusted association with changes in functional status.[46]

Aging is associated with disproportionate effects on the rate of change in ECF.[47] Therefore, ECF impairment is so common in old age as to be statistically 'normal.' Thus, although only 4% of non-institutionalized retirees may have ECF impairment at an age-specific threshold of 1.5 standard deviations below the mean, 38%[48] have impairment at a level that perfectly distinguishes patients who do, or do not have the capacity to learn to use an inhaler[37] or accurately self-assess their financial decision-making capacity.[49]

At present, MCI cases are most often distinguished from dementia solely on the basis of a CDR score. However, this measure has not been validated as a measure of disability, and may select for MCI cases which cannot be distinguished from dementia on the basis of their IADL.[50]

CAN EXECUTIVE CONTROL FUNCTION IMPAIRMENT BE OBSERVED IN THE ABSENCE OF DISABILITY?

Many studies have confirmed ECF's independent effects on functional outcomes in 'non-demented' elderly persons (Table 3.1). However, some authors fail to find significant associations, and the partial variance in functional outcomes attributable to ECF can be surprisingly small.[51] There may be many reasons for this.

First, ECF's modest independent association with functional status must be considered in the context of cognition's general failure to explain functional outcomes. Memory, attention, and verbal functions explain far less variance in functional outcomes.[51] Secondly, the association between cognition and functional outcome may be non-linear, and not amenable to linear multivariate regression techniques used by the articles in Table 3.1.[52] Thirdly, ECF is a multidimensional construct.[5] Not all 'executive' domains may be equally capable of explaining functional outcomes.[11,51] To the extent that subsets of executive functions disproportionately account for the variance in functional outcomes, they will also be particularly likely to define dementing processes. Fourthly, the association between cognition and disability may vary with the functional outcome in question. The specific disabilities indicative of dementia have never been clearly articulated. However, ECF generally explains more variance in IADL than in basic ADL, and is a particularly powerful predictor of 'higher' decision-making capacity.[35,51]

Finally, the conclusions about longitudinal processes (such as cognitive aging or dementing illness) that can be validly drawn from cross-sectional data are severely limited.[53] A growing body of longitudinal studies clearly document cognitive decline in persons who cannot be diagnosed with dementia at baseline. A few such studies include ECF measures. These generally document stronger associations with functional outcomes than the cross-sectional models presented in Table 3.1.[46,48] Non-verbal and executive measures may be particularly relevant to functional outcomes.[54–56]

IS ISOLATED EXECUTIVE CONTROL FUNCTION IMPAIRMENT A TRUE 'DEMENTIA'?

Isolated ECF impairment cannot be classified as 'dementia' by either the DSM[29] or the NINCDS.[30] However, the role of memory as the *sine qua non* of dementia's cognitive impairments can be questioned. Not only does ECF explain more variance in functional outcomes than do other cognitive domains,[51] but pathology in the CNS ROIs that subserve ECF is more strongly associated with clinical dementia than that in other ROIs.[5,17]

Recent studies suggest that ECF impairment is the one cognitive deficit that is common to dementia across diagnoses.[57–61] I have proposed the concept of (type 2) dementias 'without cortical features,' to distinguish isolated cognitive impairment from the amnestic 'cortical' dementia syndrome associated with AD.[62,63] Type 2 dementias can be discriminated from AD on the basis of simple bedside measures,[52,64,65] and have a distinct differential,[66,67] mortality,[68] and longitudinal course.[52]

Type 2 dementia is arguably an authentic dementia in that it is an acquired syndrome of disabling cognitive impairment in a clear sensorium. As such, it meets the 'California Rules' for dementia diagnosis.[69] Since other cognitive domains, notably memory impairment, contribute little variance to functional outcomes independently of ECF, the absence of memory impairment in type 2 disorders has little to say about the 'severity' of the condition (at least when judged from the perspective of its effects on functional capacity). Moreover, the demonstrable functional impairment associated with executive dyscontrol argues against the idea of 'mild' executive impairment. Indeed, the association appears causative in longitudinal analyses.[48]

Isolated executive impairment is at least as common as 'amnestic' MCI and may be much more common than clinical 'type 1' dementia.[52] Very few studies have specifically tested the prevalence of ECF impairment in the community. However, those that are available suggest a prevalence rate of 25–50% in older persons.[70,71] Almost half of these have isolated ECF impairment.[71] The differential of type 2 dementia is heterogeneous and includes many potentially reversible, non-AD conditions.[63] The label 'MCI' obscures their lack of association with AD pathology, misleads us towards inappropriate therapeutic strategies, and blinds us to their disabling cognitive declines.

CONCLUSION

ECF impairment is common in 'non-demented' populations, and may also contribute significantly to the dementia risk of 'amnestic' MCI. However, the robust specific association between ECF and disability, coupled with the close association between frontal system lesions and clinical dementia, argue against the straightforward classification of isolated ECF impairment as 'dysexecutive MCI'. Instead, this condition is worthy of consideration as an authentic dementia syndrome. In fact, ECF impairment may be essential to the clinical diagnosis of dementia, irregardless of its cause. If so, then type 2 dementia may be the most prevalent manifestation of dementing illness, albeit one which has not been well served by current dementia definitions.

Table 3.1 Published multivariate executive cognitive models of disability in 'non-demented' elderly persons

Reference	n	Subjects	Disability measure	Analysis	Covariates	Variance $(R^2)^a$
Mysiw et al[72]	38	Stroke patients	Barthel's Index	SRM	Cognitive covariates	$R^2 = 0 \times$ MMSE $R^2 = 0$ Albert's test $R^2 = 0.06 \times$ NCSE orientation $R^2 = 0.256 \times$ NCSE attention $R^2 = 0.119 \times$ NCSE repetition $R^2 = 0.102 \times$ NCSE calculations **$R^2 = 0.215 \times$ NCSE judgment** $R^2 = 0 \times$ NCSE comprehension $R^2 = 0.06 \times$ NCSE naming $R^2 = 0.06 \times$ NCSE constructions $R^2 = 0.06 \times$ NCSE memory $R^2 = 0.06 \times$ NCSE similarities
Galski et al.[73] (a)	86	Geriatric rehabilitation patients (n = 50 s/p stroke; n = 36 s/p hip fracture)	Length of stay	MR	CVA, admission FIM and cognitive covariates	$R^2 = 0 \times$ NCSE similarities $R^2 = 0 \times$ NCSE orientation **$R^2 = 0 \times$ NCSE judgment** $R^2 = 0 \times$ NCSE construction $R^2 = 0 \times$ NCSE memory
Galski et al[73] (b)	86	Geriatric rehabilitation patients (n = 50 s/p stroke; n = 36 s/p hip fracture)	Discharge FIM	MR	CVA, admission FIM and cognitive covariates	$R^2 = 0 \times$ NCSE similarities $R^2 = 0 \times$ NCSE orientation **$R^2 = 0 \times$ NCSE judgment** $R^2 = 0 \times$ NCSE construction $R^2 = 0 \times$ NCSE memory

Table 3.1 continued.

Reference	n	Subjects	Disability measure	Analysis	Covariates	Variance $(R^2)^a$
Galski et al[73] (c)	86	Geriatric rehabilitation patients ($n = 50$ s/p stroke; $n = 36$ s/p hip fracture)	Attendant care hours	MR	CVA, admission FIM and cognitive covariates	$R^2 = 0 \times$ NCSE similarities $R^2 = 0 \times$ NCSE orientation $\mathbf{R^2 = 0 \times NCSE\ judgment}$ $R^2 = 0 \times$ NCSE construction $R^2 = 0 \times$ NCSE memory
Seidel et al[74] (a)	103	Geriatric rehabilitation cases	FIM bowel control item	SRM	Total FIM and cognitive covariates	$\mathbf{R^2 = 0.053 \times mDRS\ I/P}$ $R^2 = 0 \times$ mDRS A $\mathbf{R^2 = 0 \times mDRS\ C}$ $R^2 = 0 \times$ mDRS CS $R^2 = 0 \times$ mDRS M
Seidel et al[74] (b)	103	Geriatric rehabilitation cases	FIM bladder control item	SRM	Total FIM and cognitive covariates	$\mathbf{R^2 = 0.059 \times mDRS\ I/P}$ $R^2 = 0 \times$ mDRS A $\mathbf{R^2 = 0 \times mDRS\ C}$ $R^2 = 0 \times$ mDRS CS $R^2 = 0 \times$ mDRS M
Diehl et al[75]	62	Elderly retirees	OTDL	SEM	Age, education, physical health, hearing, vision, cardiovascular health	$R^2 = 0.048 \times$ 'crystallized' intelligence $\mathbf{R^2 = 0.23 \times 'fluid'\ intelligence}$
Royall et al[76] (a)	105	Non-institutionalized retirees	HCAT Trial 1	SRM	Age, education, and cognitive covariate	$\mathbf{R^2 = 0.63 \times EXIT25}$ $R^2 = 0.08 \times$ MMSE

Table 3.1 continued.

Reference	n	Subjects	Disability measure	Analysis	Covariates	Variance (R^2)[a]
Royall et al[76] (b)	105	Non-institutionalized retirees	HCAT Trial 3	SRM	Age, education, and cognitive covariate	$R^2 = 0.05 \times EXIT25$ $R^2 = 0.67 \times MMSE$
Grigsby et al[70] (a)	1158	Community dwelling Hispanics (n = 637) and Hispanic whites (n = 521)	ADL	MR	Age, ethnicity, gender, education, CES-D, and cognitive covariate	$R^2 = 0.005 \times BDS$ $R^2 = 0 \times MMSE$
Grigsby et al[70] (b)	1158	Community dwelling Hispanics (n = 637) and non-Hispanic whites (n = 521)	IADL	MR	Age, ethnicity, gender, education, CES-D, and cognitive covariate	$R^2 = 0.014 \times BDS$ $R^2 = 0.003 \times MMSE$
Grigsby et al[70] (c)	1158	Community dwelling Hispanics (n = 637) and non-Hispanic whites (n = 521)	SAILS /dressing	MR	Age, ethnicity, gender, education, CES-D, and cognitive covariate	$R^2 = 0.029 \times BDS$ $R^2 = 0.008 \times MMSE$
Grigsby et al[70] (d)	1158	Community dwelling Hispanics (n = 637) and non-Hispanic whites (n = 521)	SAILS /eating	MR	Age, ethnicity, gender, education, CES-D, and cognitive covariate	$R^2 = 0.026 \times BDS$ $R^2 = 0.002 \times MMSE$
Grigsby et al[70] (e)	1158	Community dwelling Hispanics (n = 637) and non-Hispanic whites (n = 521)	SAILS /handling money	MR	Age, ethnicity, gender, education, CES-D, and cognitive covariate	$R^2 = 0.109 \times BDS$ $R^2 = 0.048 \times MMSE$

Table 3.1 continued.

Reference	n	Subjects	Disability measure	Analysis	Covariates	Variance (R^2)[a]
Grigsby et al[70] (f)	1158	Community dwelling Hispanics (n = 637) and non-Hispanic whites (n = 521)	SAILS /handling medications	MR	Age, ethnicity, gender, education, CES-D, and cognitive covariate	$R^2 = 0.023 \times$ BDS $R^2 = 0.053 \times$ MMSE
Rapport et al[77]	90	Traumatic injuries	Falls	MR	Age, FIM motor, and cognitive covariates	$R^2 = 0.005 \times$ WRAT–R reading $R^2 = 0.058 \times$ visual form discrimination $R^2 = 0.013 \times$ WMS–R verbal memory **$R^2 = 0.142 \times$ WCST persev errors** **$R^2 = 0.055 \times$ Stroop** $R^2 = 0.001 \times$ Letter – number span **$R^2 = 0.003 \times$ COWA**
Royall et al[34]	107	Retirees	Level of care	SMR	Age, comorbid medical conditions, medications, depressive symptoms, problem behavior, and cognitive covariate	**$R^2 = 0.48 \times$ EXIT25** $R^2 = 0.01 \times$ MMSE

Table 3.1 continued.

Reference	n	Subjects	Disability measure	Analysis	Covariates	Variance $(R^2)^a$
Binder et al[78] (a–i)	125	Community-dwelling elderly	PPT	SRM	Age	(a) $R^2 = 0.084 \times$ Trails A **(b) $R^2 = 0.04 \times$ Trails B** (c) $R^2 = 0.023 \times$ CLT time (d) $R^2 = 0.004 \times$ CLT correct (e) $R^2 = 0.048 \times$ CFT time (f) $R^2 = 0.002 \times$ CFT correct (g) $R^2 = 0.008 \times$ WAL (h) $R^2 = 0.029 \times$ DR-20 **(i) $R^2 = 0 \times$ FAS**
Carlson et al[79] (a)	406	Community-dwelling elderly women	ADL	HSRM	Age, education, race, comorbid diseases and cognitive covariates	**$R^2 = 0.01 \times$ 'executive attention'** $R^2 = 0 \times$ 'verbal memory' $R^2 = 0.01 \times$ 'spatial learning' $R^2 = 0 \times$ 'general memory'
Carlson et al[79] (b)	406	Community-dwelling elderly women	ADL	HSMR	Age, education, race, comorbid diseases, and cognitive covariates	$R^2 = 0.005 \times$ Trails A **$R^2 = 0.001 \times$ Trails B** $R^2 = 0.004 \times$ BTA $R^2 = 0.001 \times$ HAST $R^2 = 0 \times$ HVL immediate recall $R^2 = 0 \times$ HVL delayed $R^2 = 0.004 \times$ HVL recognition $R^2 = 0.008 \times$ HB errors $R^2 = 0.008 \times$ HB trials $R^2 = 0 \times$ HPB delayed object naming $R^2 = 0.005 \times$ HB delayed placement

Table 3.1   continued.

Reference	n	Subjects	Disability measure	Analysis	Covariates	Variance (R^2)[a]
Carlson et al[79] (c)	406	Community-dwelling elderly women	IADL	HSRM	Age, education, race, comorbid diseases, and cognitive covariates	$\mathbf{R^2 = 0.066 \times}$ **'executive attention'** $R^2 = 0.001 \times$ 'verbal memory' $R^2 = 0.001 \times$ 'spatial learning' $R^2 = 0.001 \times$ 'general memory'
Carlson et al[79] (d)	406	Community-dwelling elderly women	IADL	HSRM	Age, education, race, comorbid diseases, and cognitive covariates	$R^2 = 0.012 \times$ Trails A $\mathbf{R^2 = 0.02 \times}$ **Trails B** $R^2 = 0 \times$ BTA $R^2 = 0.005 \times$ HAST $R^2 = 0.002 \times$ HVL immediate recall $R^2 = 0 \times$ HVL delayed $R^2 = 0.002 \times$ HVL recognition $R^2 = 0.002 \times$ HB errors $R^2 = 0 \times$ HB trials $R^2 = 0 \times$ HPB delayed object naming $R^2 = 0 \times$ HB delayed placement
Provinciali et al[80]	83	Patients with multiple sclerosis	EDSS	HSRM	Age, mobility, timed walk, manual dexterity	$R^2 = 0 \times$ DSS $R^2 = 0 \times$ BFSRT $\mathbf{R^2 = 0 \times}$ **FAS** $\mathbf{R^2 = 0 \times}$ **WCST** $R^2 = 0 \times$ block design

Table 3.1 continued.

Reference	n	Subjects	Disability measure	Analysis	Covariates	Variance $(R^2)^a$
Cahn-Weiner et al[81] (a)	27	Community-dwelling elderly	OTAPS	HSRM	Cognitive covariates	$R^2 = 0.29 \times$ 'executive composite' $R^2 = 0 \times$ grooved pegboard $R^2 = 0.0 \times$ JLO $R^2 = 0.0 \times$ BNT $R^2 = 0.0 \times$ memory composite
Cahn-Weiner et al[81] (b)	27	Community-dwelling elderly	OTAPS	HSMR	Age, depression, and education	$R^2 = 0.19 \times$ 'executive composite'
Putzke et al[82] (a)	113	75 heart transplant candidates and 38 controls	EPT Food preparation	MR	Race, education, and cognitive covariates	$R^2 = 0.09 \times$ SILS-VOC $\mathbf{R^2 = 0.16 \times SILS\text{-}AB}$ $R^2 = 0.073 \times$ WRAT $R^2 = 0.212 \times$ PEG-D $R^2 = 0.152 \times$ PEG-ND $R^2 = 0.053 \times$ WMS-R: LM I $R^2 = 0.029 \times$ WMS-R: LM II $R^2 = 0.012 \times$ Trails A $\mathbf{R^2 = 0.212 \times Trails\ B}$ $\mathbf{R^2 = 0.012 \times CAT}$ $\mathbf{R^2 = 0.109 \times UFOV}$

Table 3.1   continued.

Reference	n	Subjects	Disability measure	Analysis	Covariates	Variance (R^2)[a]
Putzke et al[82] (b)	113	75 heart transplant candidates and 38 controls	EPT Medication	MR	Race, education, and cognitive covariates	$R^2 = 0.09 \times$ SILS-VOC $\mathbf{R^2 = 0.078 \times}$ **SILS-AB** $R^2 = 0.002 \times$ WRAT $R^2 = 0.2 \times$ PEG-D $R^2 = 0.176 \times$ PEG-ND $R^2 = 0.09 \times$ WMSR: LM I $R^2 = 0.078 \times$ WMSR: LM II $R^2 = 0.01 \times$ Trails A $\mathbf{R^2 = 0.152 \times}$ **Trails B** $\mathbf{R^2 = 0.053 \times}$ **CAT** $\mathbf{R^2 = 0.058 \times}$ **UFOV**
Putzke et al[82] (c)	113	75 heart transplant candidates and 38 controls	EPT Phone use	MR	Race, education, and cognitive covariates	$R^2 = 0.203 \times$ SILS-VOC $\mathbf{R^2 = 0.16 \times}$ **SILS-AB** $R^2 = 0.109 \times$ WRAT $R^2 = 0.171 \times$ PEG-D $R^2 = 0.053 \times$ PEG-ND $R^2 = 0.026 \times$ WMS-R: LM I $R^2 = 0.014 \times$ WMS-R: LM II $R^2 = 0.06 \times$ Trails A $\mathbf{R^2 = 0.123 \times}$ **Trails B** $\mathbf{R^2 = 0.02 \times}$ **CAT** $\mathbf{R^2 = 0.063 \times}$ **UFOV**

Table 3.1 continued.

Reference	n	Subjects	Disability measure	Analysis	Covariates	Variance (R^2)[a]
Putzke et al[82] (d)	113	75 heart transplant candidates and 38 controls	EPT Shopping	MR	Race, education, and cognitive covariates	$R^2 = 0.068 \times$ SILS-VOC **$R^2 = 0.096 \times$ SILS-AB** $R^2 = 0.012 \times$ WRAT $R^2 = 0.078 \times$ PEG-D $R^2 = 0.152 \times$ PEG-ND $R^2 = 0.029 \times$ WMS-R: LM I $R^2 = 0.01 \times$ WMS-R: LM II $R^2 = 0.02 \times$ Trails A **$R^2 = 0.116 \times$ Trails B** **$R^2 = 0.048 \times$ CAT** **$R^2 = 0.137 \times$ UFOV**
Putzke et al[82] (e)	113	75 heart transplant candidates and 38 controls	EPT Finance	MR	Race, education, and cognitive covariates	$R^2 = 0.053 \times$ SILS-VOC **$R^2 = 0.13 \times$ SILS-AB** $R^2 = 0.04 \times$ WRAT $R^2 = 0.014 \times$ PEG-D $R^2 = 0.036 \times$ PEG-ND $R^2 = 0.023 \times$ WMS-R: LM I $R^2 = 0.005 \times$ WMS-R: LM II $R^2 = 0 \times$ Trails A **$R^2 = 0.109 \times$ Trails B** **$R^2 = 0.068 \times$ CAT** **$R^2 = 0.023 \times$ UFOV**

Table 3.1   continued.

Reference	n	Subjects	Disability measure	Analysis	Covariates	Variance $(R^2)^a$
Putzke et al[82] (f)	113	75 heart transplant candidates and 38 controls	EPT Household chores	MR	Race, education, and cognitive covariates	$R^2 = 0.185 \times$ SILS-VOC $\mathbf{R^2 = 0.25 \times}$ **SILS-AB** $R^2 = 0.084 \times$ WRAT $R^2 = 0.048 \times$ PEG-D $R^2 = 0.078 \times$ PEG-ND $R^2 = 0.032 \times$ WMS-R: LM I $R^2 = 0.008 \times$ WMS-R: LM II $R^2 = 0.003 \times$ Trails A $\mathbf{R^2 = 0.203 \times}$ **Trails B** $\mathbf{R^2 = 0.048 \times}$ **CAT** $\mathbf{R^2 = 0.123 \times}$ **UFOV**
Putzke et al[82] (g)	113	75 heart transplant candidates and 38 controls	EPT Transportation	MR	Race, education, and cognitive covariates	$R^2 = 0.23 \times$ SILS-VOC $\mathbf{R^2 = 0.23 \times}$ **SILS-AB** $R^2 = 0.102 \times$ WRAT $R^2 = 0.026 \times$ PEG-D $R^2 = 0.04 \times$ PEG-ND $R^2 = 0.068 \times$ WMS-R: LM I $R^2 = 0.026 \times$ WMS-R: LM II $R^2 = 0.026 \times$ Trails A $\mathbf{R^2 = 0.203 \times}$ **Trails B** $\mathbf{R^2 = 0.04 \times}$ **CAT** $\mathbf{R^2 = 0.096 \times}$ **UFOV**

Table 3.1   continued.

Reference	n	Subjects	Disability measure	Analysis	Covariates	Variance (R^2)[a]
Royall et al[34] (a)	561	Well elderly	IADLs	MR	Age, medications, caregiver, and cognitive covariates	$R^2 = 0.0256 \times$ CLOX2 $R^2 = 0.0256 \times$ EXIT25 $R^2 = 0 \times$ MMSE $R^2 = 0 \times$ CLOX1
Dymek et al[35] (a)	40	$n = 20$ patients with Parkinson's disease $n = 20$ controls	CCTI: evidencing a choice	SRM	Cognitive covariates	$R^2 = 0 \times$ mDRS A $R^2 = 0.55 \times$ mDRS M $R^2 = 0 \times$ EXIT25 $R^2 = 0 \times$ WAIS-R: C
Dymek et al[35] (b)	40	$n = 20$ patients with Parkinson's disease $n = 20$ controls	CCTI: rational reasons	SRM	Cognitive covariates	$R^2 = 0 \times$ mDRS A $R^2 = 0 \times$ WMS-R: LM II $R^2 = 0.45 \times$ EXIT25 $R^2 = 0 \times$ Trails B
Dymek et al[35] (c)	40	$n = 20$ patients with Parkinson's disease $n = 20$ controls	CCTI: understanding treatment	SRM	Cognitive covariates	$R^2 = 0 \times$ WMS-R: LM II $R^2 = 0.12 \times$ mDRS M $R^2 = 0.56 \times$ EXIT25 $R^2 = 0 \times$ WAIS-R: C
Bell-McGinty et al[83]	50	Community elderly	ILS-FSS	MR	Cognitive covariates	$R^2 = 0.203 \times$ Trails B $R^2 = 0.014 \times$ COWA $R^2 = 0 \times$ mDRS: I/P $R^2 = 0.014 \times$ MPT $R^2 = 0.073 \times$ WCST

Table 3.1 continued.

Reference	n	Subjects	Disability measure	Analysis	Covariates	Variance (R^2)[a]
Beloosesky et al[84]	153	Rehabilitation patients with hip fractures	ΔFIM (self-care)	MR	Age, gender, Katz ADL, baseline FIM	$R^2 = 0.0 \times$ MMSE
Cahn-Weiner et al[85] (a)	30	Well community elderly	OTAPS	MR	Cognitive covariates	$R^2 = 0.26 \times$ Trails B $R^2 = 0.0 \times$ COWA $R^2 = 0.0 \times$ WCST: persev errors
Cahn-Weiner et al[85] (b)	30	Well community elderly	IADLs	MR	Cognitive covariates	$R^2 = 0.20 \times$ Trails B $R^2 = 0.14 \times$ COWA $R^2 = 0.0 \times$ WCST: persev errors
Cahn-Weiner et al[85] (c)	30	Well community elderly	ADLs	MR	Cognitive covariates	$R^2 = 0.0 \times$ Trails B $R^2 = 0.0 \times$ COWA $R^2 = 0.0 \times$ WCST: persev errors
Giovannetti et al[86] (a)	51	Memory-impaired outpatients	MLAT-S total	MR	Cognitive covariates	$R^2 = 0.28 \times$ MMSE $R^2 = 0 \times$ 'executive' composite $R^2 = 0 \times$ 'semantic' composite
Giovannetti et al[86] (b)	51	Memory-impaired outpatients	MLAT-S ommission errors	MR	Cognitive covariates	$R^2 = 0.32 \times$ MMSE $R^2 = 0 \times$ 'executive' composite $R^2 = 0 \times$ 'semantic' composite
Giovannetti et al[86] (c)	51	Memory-impaired outpatients	MLAT-S omission errors	MR	Cognitive covariates	$R^2 = 0 \times$ MMSE $R^2 = 0 \times$ 'executive' composite $R^2 = 0 \times$ 'semantic' composite

Table 3.1 continued.

Reference	n	Subjects	Disability measure	Analysis	Covariates	Variance $(R^2)^a$
Mayer et al[87] (a)	113	Patients with subarachnoid hemorrhage	mRS	HSRM	Age, gender, race, education, English fluency, depressive symptoms, and cognitive covariates	$R^2 = 0.093 \times$ TICS $R^2 = 0 \times$ visual memory $R^2 = 0 \times$ verbal memory $R^2 = 0 \times$ reaction time $R^2 = 0 \times$ motor function **$R^2 = 0 \times$ executive function** $R^2 = 0 \times$ visuospatial function $R^2 = 0 \times$ language function
Mayer et al[87] (b)	113	Patients with subarachnoid hemorrhage	SIP-physical	HSMR	Age, gender, race, education, English fluency, depressive symptoms, and cognitive covariates	$R^2 = 0.08 \times$ TICS $R^2 = 0 \times$ visual memory $R^2 = 0 \times$ verbal memory $R^2 = 0 \times$ reaction time $R^2 = 0.027 \times$ motor function **$R^2 = 0 \times$ executive function** $R^2 = 0 \times$ visuospatial function $R^2 = 0 \times$ language function
Mayer et al[87] (c)	113	Patients with subarachnoid hemorrhage	SIP-psychosocial	HSMR	Age, gender, race, education, English fluency, depressive symptoms, and cognitive covariates	$R^2 = 0.034 \times$ TICS $R^2 = 0 \times$ visual memory $R^2 = 0 \times$ verbal memory $R^2 = 0 \times$ reaction time $R^2 = 0 \times$ motor function **$R^2 = 0 \times$ executive function** $R^2 = 0.029 \times$ visuospatial function $R^2 = 0 \times$ language function

Table 3.1 continued.

Reference	n	Subjects	Disability measure	Analysis	Covariates	Variance (R^2)[a]
Mayer et al[87] (d)	113	Patients with subarachnoid hemorrhage	SIP-total	HSMR	Age, gender, race, education, English fluency, depressive symptoms, and cognitive covariates	$R^2 = 0.051 \times$ TICS $R^2 = 0 \times$ visual memory $R^2 = 0 \times$ verbal memory $R^2 = 0 \times$ reaction time $R^2 = 0 \times$ motor function **$R^2 = 0 \times$ executive function** $R^2 = 0 \times$ visuospatial function $R^2 = 0 \times$ language function
Mok et al[88] (a)	117	75 geriatric stroke patients with 'small vessel disease' 42 controls	BI	MR	Age, education, NIHSS, pre-stroke IQCODE, stroke history, heart disease, silent infarcts, WMC, and cognitive covariates	$R^2 = 0\times$ MMSE **$R^2 = 0 \times$ mDRS: I/P** $R^2 = 0 \times$ ADAS-cog
Mok et al[88] (b)	117	75 geriatric stroke patients with 'small vessel disease' 42 controls	IADL	MR	Age, education, NIHSS, pre-stroke IQCODE, stroke history, heart disease, silent infarcts, WMC, and cognitive covariates	$R^2 = 0 \times$ MMSE **$R^2 = 0.139 \times$ mDRS: I/P** $R^2 = 0 \times$ ADAS-cog
Royall et al[48]	457	Retirees	ΔIADLs	MR	Age, level, IADL, comorbid diseases, level of care, and cognitive covariates	**$R^2 = 0 \times$ EXIT25** **$R^2 = 0.33 \times$ ΔEXIT25**

Table 3.1 continued.

Reference	n	Subjects	Disability measure	Analysis	Covariates	Variance (R^2)[a]
Rapp et al[89] (a)	299	n = 96 institutionalized and n = 192 non-institutionalized retirees	CDR ADL ratings	HSRM	Age, gender, education, dementia status, level of care, and cognitive covariates	$R^2 = 0.039 \times$ MMSE $R^2 = 0.002 \times$ ECF/speed factor $R^2 = 0.016 \times$ ECF factor $R^2 = 0 \times$ memory factor
Rapp et al[89] (b)	299	n = 96 institutionalized and n = 192 non-institutionalized retirees	CDR ADL ratings	HSMR	Age, gender, education, dementia status, level of care, and cognitive covariates	$R^2 = 0 \times$ MMSE $R^2 = 0.001 \times$ ECF/speed factor $R^2 = 0.04 \times$ ECF factor $R^2 = 0.003 \times$ memory factor
Royall et al[46]	457	Retirees	ΔIADLs	MR	Age, level, IADL, comorbid diseases, level of care, and cognitive covariates	$R^2 = 0.033 \times$ EXIT25 $R^2 = 0.001 \times$ CVLT $R^2 = 0.276 \times$ ΔEXIT25 $R^2 = 0.017 \times$ ΔCVLT
Royall et al[55] (a)	457	Retirees	ΔIADLs	MR	Age, level, IADL, comorbid diseases, level of care, and cognitive covariates	$R^2 = 0.047 \times$ EXIT25 $R^2 = 0.039 \times$ WCAT $R^2 = 0.276 \times$ ΔEXIT25 $R^2 = 0.019 \times$ ΔWCAT
Royall et al[55] (b)	457	Retirees	ΔIADLs	MR	Age, level, IADL, comorbid diseases, level of care, and cognitive covariates	$R^2 = 0.025 \times$ EXIT25 $R^2 = 0.072 \times$ WCST: CNPT $R^2 = 0.311 \times$ ΔEXIT25 $R^2 = 0.042 \times$ ΔWCST: CNPT

Table 3.1 continued.

[a] Variance (R2) explained by disability labeled factor in factor analytic models, or variance in regression models of a disability measure that is explained by its significant cognitive correlates. Univariate and partial correlations were squared to determine R^2 when variance was not specifically reported. Executive measures in bold type.

ADAS-cog = Alzheimer's Disease Assessment Scale: Cognitive subscale; ADLs = Activities of Daily Living; BDS = Behavioral Dyscontrol Scale; BFSRT = Buschke–Fuld selective remind test; BI = ; BNT = Boston Naming Test; BTA = Brief Test of Attention; CAT = Short Category Test; CCT1 = Capacity to Consent to Treatment Instrument; CDR = Clinical Dementia Rating scale; CES–D = Clinical Evaluation of Depression; CFT = ; CLOX = An Executive Clock-drawing Task; CLT = ; COWA = Controlled Oral Word Association; CVA = cerebrovascular accident or 'stroke'; CVLT = California Verbal Learning Test; ∆CVLT = change in CVLT; DR-20 = 20 minute Delayed Recall; EDSS = ; ECF = Executive Control Function; EPT = Everyday Performance Test; EXIT25 = Executive Interview; ∆EXIT25 = change in EXIT25 scores; FA = factor analysis; FAS = FAS verbal fluency; FIM = Functional Independence Measure; ∆FIM = change in FIM; GCC = general cognition construct; GCCS = General Cognitive Composite Score; HAST = Hopkins Attention Screening Test; HB = Hopkins (peg) board; HCAT = Hopkins Competency Assessment Test; HSRM = hierarchical stepwise regression model; HPB = ; HVL = Hopkins Verbal Learning test; IADLs = Instrumental Activities of Daily Living; ∆IADLs = longitudinal change in IADLs; IQCODE = Informant Questionnaire on Cognitive Decline in the Elderly; JLO = Judgment Line Orientation; mDRS = Mattis Dementia Rating Scale (A = attention, CS = constructions, C = conceptualization; I/P = initiation/perseveration; M = memory); MLAT-S = Multi-level Action Test (short version); MMSE = Mini-Mental State Examination; MPT = Manual Postures Test; MR = multiple regression; mRS = modified Rankin Scale; NCSE = Neurobehavioral Cognitive Status Examination; NIHSS = National Institutes of Health Stroke Severity; OTAPS = ; OTDL = Observational Tasks of Daily Living; PADL = Physical ADLs; PEG = Grooved Pegboard, D = dominant hand, ND = non-dominant; SAILS = Structured Assessment of Independent Living Skills; SILS = Shipley Institute of Living Scale, AB = abstraction, VOC = vocabulary; SIP = Sickness Impact Profile; SRM = (unforced) stepwise regression model; TICS = Telephone Interview of Cognitive Status; UFOV = Useful Field of View; WAIS = Weschler Adult Intelligence Scale (-R = Revised): Block = Block Design, C = Conceptualization, SIM = Similarities; WAL = Weschler Associate Learning; WCAT = categories completed on the Wisconsin Card Sorting Task; ∆WCAT = change in WCAT; WCST = Wisconsin Card Sorting Task: persev errors = perseverative errors, CNPT = conceptualization, CNPT = change in WCST: CPT; WMS = Weschler Memory Scale (- R = Revised): LM = Logical Memory, WRAT = Wide Range Achievement Test.

REFERENCES

1. Petersen RC, Smith GE, Waring SC, et al. Mild cognitive impairment: clinical characterization and outcome. Arch Neurol 1999;56:303–308.

2. Petersen RC, Stevens JC, Ganguli M, et al. Practice parameter: early detection of dementia: mild cognitive impairment (an evidence-based review). Report of the Quality Standards Subcommittee of the American Academy of Neurology. Neurology 2001;56:1133–1142.

3. Busse A, Bischkopf J, Riedel-Heller SG, Angemeyer MC. Subclassifications for mild cognitive impairment: prevalence and predicitive validity. Psychol Med 2003;33:1029–1038.

4. Thompson PM, Hayshi KM, de Zubicaray G, et al. Dynamics of gray matter loss in Alzheimer's disease. J Neurosci 2003;23, 994–1005.

5. Royall DR, Lauterbach EC, Cummings JL, et al. Executive control function: a review of its promise and challenges to clinical research. A report from the Committee on Research of the American Neuropsychiatric Association. J Neuropsychiatry Clin Neurosci 2002;14:377–405.

6. DeKosky ST, Scheff SW. Synapse loss in frontal cortex biopsies in Alzheimer's disease: correlation with cognitive severity. Ann Neurol 1990;27:457–464.

7. Geddes JW, Snowdon DA, Soultanian NS, et al. Braak Stages III–IV of Alzheimer's related neuropathology are associated with mild memory loss. Stages V–VI are associated with dementia: Findings from the Nun Study. J Neuropathol Exp Neurol 1996;55:617.

8. Royall DR, Palmer R, Mulroy A, et al. Pathological determinants of the transition to clinical dementia in Alzheimer's disease. Exp Aging Res 2002;28:143–162.

9. Hughes CP, Berg L, Danziger WL, Coben LA, Martin RL. A new clinical scale for the staging of dementia. Br J Psychiatr 1982;140:566–572.

10. Pandya DN, Yeterain FH. Comparison of prefrontal architecture and connections. Phil Trans Royal Soc London, B: Biol Sci 1998;351:1423–1432.

11. Royall DR, Chiodo LK, Polk M. Executive dyscontrol in normal aging: Normative data, factor structure, and clinical correlates. In Brust JCM, Fahn S, eds. Current neurology and neuroscience reports. Philadelphia. Current Science; 2003;6:487–493

12. Reiman RM, Caselli RJ, Yun LS, et al. Preclinical evidence of Alzheimer's disease in persons homozygous for the ε4 allele for apolipoprotein E. N Engl J Med 1996;334:752–758.

13. Snowdon DA, Grenier LH, Mortimer JA, et al. Brain infarction and the clinical expression of Alzheimer disease. The Nun Study. JAMA 1997;277: 813–817.

14. Goulding JM, Signorini DF, Chatterjee S, et al. Inverse relation between Braak stage and cerebrovascular pathology in Alzheimer predominant dementia. J Neurol Neurosurg Psychiatry 1999;67:654–657.

15. White L, Petrovitch H, Hardman J, et al. Cerebrovascular pathology and dementia in autopsied Honolulu-Asia Aging Study Participants. Annals N Y Acad Sci 2002;977:9–23.

16. Royall DR. The new 'silent' epidemic. J Am Geriatr Soc 2004;52:1212–1213.

17. Zekry D, Duyckaerts C, Belmin J, et al. The vascular lesions in vascular and mixed dementia: the weight of functional neuroanatomy. Neurobiol Aging 2003;24:213–219.

18. Kelly PA, McCulloch J. Extrastriatal circuits activated by intrastriatal muscimol: a [^{14}C]2-deoxyglucose investigation. Brain Res 1984;292:357–366

19. Román GC, Royall DR. A diagnostic dilemma: is 'Alzheimer's dementia' Alzheimer's disease, vascular demen-

tia, or both? Lancet Neurol 2004;3:141.

20. Lowenstein DA, Ownby R, Schram L, et al. An evaluation of the NINCDS-ADRDA neuropsychological criteria for the assessment of Alzheimer's disease: a confirmatory factor analysis of single versus multi-factor models. J Clin Exp Neuropsychol 2001;23:274–284.

21. Willis SL, Allen-Burge R, Dolan MM, et al. Everyday problem solving among individuals with Alzheimer's disease. Gerontologist 1998;38:569–577.

22. Chen ST, Sultzer DC, Hinkin CH, Mahler ME, Cummings JL. Executive dysfunction in Alzheimer's disease: association with neuropsychiatric symptoms and functional impairment. J Neuropsychiatry Clin Neurosci 1998;10:426–432.

23. Boyle PA, Malloy PF, Salloway S, et al. Executive dysfunction and apathy predict functional impairment in Alzheimer disease. Am J Geriatr Psychiatry 2003;11:214–221.

24. Marson DC, Chatterjee A, Ingram KK, Harrell LE. Toward a neurologic model of competency. Cognitive predictors of capacity to consent in Alzheimer's disease using the three different legal standards. Neurology 1998;46:666–672.

25. Marson DC, Cody HA, Ingram KK, Harrell LE. Neuropsychological predictors of competency in Alzheimer's disease using a rational reasons legal standard. Arch Neurol 1995;52:955–959.

26. Nagahama Y, Okina T, Suzuki N, et al. Factor structure of a modified version of the Wisconsin card sorting test: an analysis of executive deficit in Alzheimer's disease and mild cognitive impairment. Dement Geriatr Cogn Disord 2003;16:103–112.

27. Ready RE, Ott BR, Grace J, Cahn-Weiner DA. Apathy and executive dysfunction in mild cognitive impairment and Alzheimer disease. Am J Geriatr Psychiatry 2003;11:222–228.

28. Royall DR. The 'Alzheimerization' of dementia research. J Am Geriatr Soc 2003;51:277–278.

29. American Psychiatric Association. Diagnostic and statistical manual of mental disorders, 4th ed. Washington, DC: American Psychiatric Association; 1994

30. McKhann G, Drachman D, Folstein M, et al. Clinical diagnosis of Alzheimer's disease: report of the NINCDS-ADRDA Work Group under the auspices of the Department of Health and Human Services Task Force on Alzheimer's disease. Neurology 1984;34:939–944.

31. Schillerstrom JE, Royall DR, Stern SL, Deuter MS, Wyatt R. Prevalence of executive impairment in patients seen by a psychiatry consult-liaison service. Psychosomatics 2003;44;290–297.

32. Royall DR, Mahurin RK, Gray K. Bedside assessment of executive cognitive impairment: the executive interview. J Am Geriatr Soc 1992;40:1221–1226.

33. Royall DR, Chiodo LK, Polk MJ. Correlates of disability among elderly retirees with "sub-clinical" cognitive impairment. J Gerontol Med Sci 2000:55A:M541–546.

34. Royall DR, Cabello M, Polk MJ. Executive dyscontrol: an important factor affecting the level of care received by elderly retirees. J Am Geriatr Soc 1998;46:1519–1524.

35. Dymek MP, Atchison P, Harrell L, Marson DC. Competency to consent to medical treatment in cognitively impaired patients with Parkinson's. Neurology 2001;56:17–24.

36. Mann LS, Westlake T, Wise TN, et al. Executive functioning and compliance in HIV patients. Psychol Rep 1999;84:319–322.

37. Allen SC, Jain M, Ragab S, Malik N. Acquisition and short-term retention of inhaler techniques require intact executive function in elderly subjects. Age Ageing 2003;32:299–302.

38. Kelly C, Sharkey V, Morrison G, Allardyce J, McCreadie G. Cognitive function in a catchment-area-based population of patients with schizophrenia. Br J Psychiatry 2000;177: 348–353.

37. Allen SC, Jain M, Ragab S, Malik N. Acquisition and short-term retention of inhaler techniques require intact executive function in elderly subjects. Age Ageing 2003;32:299–302.

38. Kelly C, Sharkey V, Morrison G, Allardyce J, McCreadie G. Cognitive function in a catchment-area-based population of patients with schizophrenia. Br J Psychiatry 2000;177: 348–353.

39. Fuss M, Boersma M, Sheriff H, Royall DR. Prevalence of executive control function (ECF) impairment among patients referred for radiotherapy. Radiother Oncol 2002;64:S154.

40. Schillerstrom JE, Horton MS, Earthman BS, et al. Prevalence, course, and risk factors for executive impairment in patients hospitalized on a general medicine service. Psychosomatics in press.

41. Royall DR, Chiodo LK, Polk MJ. Prevalence and severity of executive cognitive impairment among diabetic outpatients. Gerontologist 1999;39: (Supp 1):470.

42. Folstein M, Folstein S, McHugh PR. 'Mini Mental State': a practical method for grading the cognitive state of patients for the clinician. J Psychiatric Res 1975;12:189–198.

43. Royall DR, Chiodo LK, Polk MJ. Misclassification is likely in the assessment of mild cognitive impairment. Neuroepidemiology 2004;23: 185–191.

44. Royall DR, Chiodo LK, Polk MJ, Jaramillo CJ. Severe dysosmia is specifically associated with Alzheimer-like memory deficits in non-demented elderly retirees. Neuroepidemiology 2002;21:68–73.

45. Hofer SM, Christensen H, Mackinnon AJ, Korten AE, Jorm AF. Change in cognitive functioning associated with ApoE genotype in a community sample of older adults. Psychol Aging 2002;17:194–208.

46. Royall DR, Palmer R, Chiodo LK, Polk MJ. Executive control mediates memory's association with change in instrumental activities of daily living: the Freedom House Study. J Am Geriatr Soc 2005;53:11–17.

47. Royall DR, Vicioso B. Aging overview. In: Aminoff M, Daroff RB, eds. Encyclopedia of the neurological sciences, Vol. 1. San Diego: Academic Press; 2003:53–57.

48. Royall DR, Palmer R, Chiodo LK, Polk MJ. Declining executive control in normal aging predicts change in functional status: the Freedom House Study. J Am Geriatr Soc 2004;52: 346–352.

49. Fan E, Royall DR, Chiodo L, Polk MJ, Mouton C. Insight into financial capacity in non-institutionalized retirees. J Am Geriatr Soc 2003; 51(s4):S80.

50. Albert SM, Michaels K, Padilla M, et al. Functional significance of mild cognitive impairment in elderly patients without a dementia diagnosis. Am J Geriatr Psychiatry 1999;7: 213–220.

51. Royall DR, Malloy P, Lauterbach EC, Kaufer DI, and the Committee on Research of the American Neuropsychiatric Association. The cognitive correlates of functional status: a review from the Committee on Research of the American Neuropsychiatric Association J Neuropsychiatry Clin Neurosci in press.

52. Royall DR, Espino DV, Polk M, Palmer R, Markides KS. Prevalence and patterns of executive impairment in community dwelling Mexican Americans: results from the Hispanic EPESE Study. Int J Geriatr Psychiatry, 2004; b;19:926–934.

53. Kraemer HC, Yesavage JA, Taylor JL, Kupfer D. How can we learn about developmental processes from cross-

sectional studies, or can we? Am J Psychiatry 2000;157:163–171.

54. Artero S, Touchon J, Ritchie K. Disability and mild cognitive impairment: a longitudinal population-based study. Int J Geriatr Psychiatry 2001;16:1092–1097.

55. Royall DR, Palmer R, Chiodo LK, Polk MJ. Wisconsin Card Sort performance fails to predict change in functional status in old age: the Freedom House Study J Clin Exp Neuropsychology in press.

56. Royall DR, Palmer R, Chiodo LK, Polk MJ. Normal rates of cognitive change in successful aging: the Freedom House Study. J Int Neuropsychol Soc in press.

57. Bernard BA, Wilson RS, Gilley DW, et al. The dementia of Binswanger's disease and Alzheimer's disease. Neuropsychiatry Neuropsychol Behavioral Neurol 1994 7:30–35.

58. Lange KW, Shahakian BJ, Quinn NP, Marsden TW. Comparison of executive and visuospatial memory function in Huntington's disease and dementia of the Alzheimer type matched for degree of dementia. J Neurol Neurosurg Psychiatry 1995;58: 598–606.

59. Paulsen JS, Butters N, Sadek JR, et al. Distinct cognitive profiles of cortical and subcortical dementia in advanced illness. Neurology 1995;45:951–956.

60. Voss SE, Bullock RA. Executive function: The core feature of dementia? Dement Geriatr Cogn Disord 2004; 18:207–216.

61. De Jager CA, Hogervorst E, Combrinck M, Budge MM. Sensitivity and specificity of neuropsychological tests for mild cognitive impairment, vascular cognitive impairment and Alzheimer's disease. Psychol Med 2003;33:1039–1050.

62. Royall DR, Polk MJ. Dementias that present with and without posterior cortical features: an important clinical distinction. J Am Geriatr Soc 1998; 46:98–105.

63. Royall DR. Executive cognitive impairment: a novel perspective on dementia. Neuroepidemiology 2000;19:293–299.

64. Royall DR, Mahurin RK, Cornell J, Gray K. Bedside assessment of dementia type using the Qualitative Evaluation of Dementia (QED). Neuropsychiatry Neuropsychol Behavioral Neurol 1993;6:235–244.

65. Royall DR. Bedside assessment of vascular dementia. In Gauthier S, Erkinjuntti T, eds. Vascular cognitive impairment. London: Martin Dunitz Ltd; 2002: 307–322.

66. Royall DR, Mahurin RK, Cornell JC. Bedside assessment of frontal degeneration: distinguishing Alzheimer's disease from non-Alzheimer's cortical dementia. Exp Aging Res 1994;20:95–103.

67. Royall DR, Mahurin RK, Cornell J. Effect of depression on dementia presentation: qualitative assessment with the Qualitative Evaluation of Dementia (QED). J Geriatr Psychiatry Neurol 1995;8:4–11.

68. Royall DR, Palmer R, Chiodo LK, Polk MJ. Decline in learning ability best predicts future dementia type: the Freedom House Study. Exp Aging Res 2003;29:385–406.

69. Cummings JL, Benson DF, LoVerme S Jr. Reversible dementia: illustrative cases, definition, and review. JAMA 1980;243:2434–2439.

70. Grigsby J, Kaye K, Baxter J, Shetterly SM, Hamman RF. Executive cognitive abilities and functional status among community-dwelling older persons in the San Luis Valley Health and Aging Study. J Am Geriatr Soc 1998; 46:590–596.

71. Royall DR. The "subsyndromal" syndromes of aging. J Am Geriatr Soc. 2004;52:463–465.

72. Mysiw WJ, Beegan JG, Gatens PF. Prospective cognitive assessment of stroke patients before inpatient rehabilitation. The relationship of the Neurobehavioral Cognitive Status

Examination to functional improvement. Am J Phys Med Rehabil 1989;68:168–171.

73. Galski T, Bruno RL, Zorowitz R, Walker J. Predicting length of stay, functional outcome and aftercare in the rehabilitation of stroke patients. The dominant role of higher-order cognition. Stroke 1993;24:1794–1800.

74. Seidel GK, Millis ST, Lichtenberg PA, Dijkers M. Predicting bowel and bladder incontinence from cognitive status in geriatric rehabilitation patients. Arch Phys Med Rehabil 1994;75:590–593.

75. Diehl M, Willis SL, Schiae KW. Everyday problem solving in older adults: observational assessment and cognitive correlates. Psychol Aging 1995;10:478–491.

76. Royall DR, Cordes J, Polk M. Executive control and the comprehension of medical information by elderly retirees. Exp Aging Res 1997;23:301–313.

77. Rapport LJ, Hanks RA, Millis SR, Deshpande SA. Executive functioning and predictors of falls in the rehabilitation setting. Arch Phys Med Rehabil 1998;79:629–633.

78. Binder EF, Storandt M, Birge SJ. The relation between psychometric test performance and physical performance in older adults. J Gerontol A Biol Sci Med Sci 1999;54:M428–432.

79. Carlson ML, Fried LP, Xue QL, et al. Association between executive attention and physical function performance in community-dwelling older women. J Gerontol B Psychol Sci Soc Sci 1999;54:S262–270.

80. Provinciali L, Ceravolo MG, Bartolini M, Logullo F, Danni M. A multidimensional assessment of multiple sclerosis: relationships between disability domains. Acta Neurol Scand 1999;100:156-162.

81. Cahn-Weiner DA, Malloy PF, Boyle PA, Marran M, Salloway S. Prediction of functional status from neuropsycho-logical tests in community-dwelling elderly individuals. Clin Neuropsychol 2000;14:187–195.

82. Putzke JD, Williams MA, Daniel FJ. Activities of daily living among heart transplant candidates: neuropsychological and cardiac function predictors. J Heart Lung Transplant 2000;19:995–1006.

83. Bell-McGinty S, Podell K, Franzen M, Baird AD, Williams MJ. Standard measures of executive function in predicting instrumental activities of daily living in older adults. Int J Geriatr Psychiatry 2002;17:828–834.

84. Beloosesky Y, Grinblat J, Epelboym B, et al. Functional gain of hip fracture patients in different cognitive and functional groups. Clin Rehabil 2002;16:321–328.

85. Cahn-Weiner DA, Boyle PA, Malloy PF. Tests of executive function predict instrumental activities of daily living in community-dwelling older individuals. Appl Neuropsychol 2002;9:187–191.

86. Giovanetti T, Libon DJ, Boxbaum LJ, Schwartz MF. Naturalistic action impairments in dementia. Neuropsychologia 2002;40:1220–1232.

87. Mayer SA, Kreiter KT, Copeland D, et al. Global and domain-specific cognitive impairment and outcome after subarachnoid hemorrhage. Neurology 2002;59:1750–1758.

88. Mok VC, Wong A, Lam WW, et al. Cognitive impairment and functional outcome after stroke associated with small vessel disease. J Neurol Neurosurg Psychiatry 2004;75:560–566.

89. Rapp MA, Schnaider-Berri M, Schmeidler J, et al. Relationship of neuropsychological performance to functional status in nursing home residents and community-dwelling older adults. Am J Geriatr Psychiatry 2005;13:450–459.

4

Glycosaminoglycan mimetics in Alzheimer's disease

Francine Gervais, Denis Garceau, Paul S Aisen, and Serge Gauthier

INTRODUCTION

Amyloid beta (Aβ) protein forms fibrillar deposits and organizes in the central nervous system as senile plaques. Plaques are one of the core neuropathologic hallmarks of Alzheimer's disease (AD). The amyloid cascade hypothesis proposes that Aβ is causally related to the neurodegeneration associated with AD and is considered a promising target for the development of a disease-modifying therapeutic approach for the disease. The severity of the disease correlates better with the presence of soluble oligomeric forms of Aβ rather than with the presence of amyloid deposits.[1,2] The oligomers have been shown to be highly neurotoxic.[2] Reducing the oligomerization process and inhibiting Aβ fibril formation may favor the metabolic clearance of Aβ and prevent the neurotoxicity and inflammation associated with oligomerization and senile plaque formation.

The conversion of soluble to fibrillary Aβ is a nucleation-dependent process[3,4] influenced by Aβ concentration, pH, and the presence of nucleation seeds such as proteoglycans and apolipoproteins. Interfering in the association of Aβ with proteoglycans has been shown to inhibit the formation of Aβ fibrils and may lead to the reduction of senile plaques by controlling the earliest stage of the amyloidogenic process.

Proteoglycans bind to several types of amyloidogenic proteins. The glycosaminoglycan (GAG) chain of these proteoglycans appears to be involved in the pathophysiology of amyloid by inducing and promoting conformational transitions in the amyloidogenic protein.[5] In AD, several types of proteoglycans associate with fibrillary Aβ in amyloid plaques and with neurofibrillary tangles.[6,7] The interactions of Aβ with proteoglycans are mainly mediated through the binding of the highly sulfated GAG chains to Aβ. In this way, the multiple and complex GAG moieties of the proteoglycans bind to amyloidogenic proteins, promote fibrillogenesis, and stabilize fibrils. Moreover, binding of GAGs to Aβ protects fibrils from proteolytic degradation and attenuates Aβ-induced neurotoxicity.[4,8] GAGs exert their fibrillogenesis-promoting effect through their binding to specific sites within amyloid proteins. GAG binding to Aβ between two neighboring protofilaments would stabilize the tertiary structure of Aβ protein, acting as a scaffold for the assembly of fibrils.[4,9]

A series of low molecular weight (MW) charged non-carbohydrate compounds have been developed to mimic the anionic properties of GAGs and are, therefore, referred to as 'functional GAG mimetics'. These compounds have been tested for their ability to block the fibrillogenesis of a number of different amyloidogenic proteins, such as AA (amyloid A), Aβ, and IAPP (islet-associated polypeptide). GAG mimetics have been shown to block the development of AA amyloid in vivo using animal models of secondary amyloidosis.[10,11] A similar approach using low-MW heparin has been reported to inhibit development of AA amyloidosis in mice.[12] GAG mimetics were found to prevent the binding of heparan sulfate to Aβ in vitro and to interfere in heparan sulfate-accelerated Aβ fibrillogenesis. Moreover, these compounds have been shown to protect primary neuronal cells against $A\beta_{40}$-induced toxicity.[13] To date, GAG mimetics exhibiting anti-amyloid activities appear to be specific for each amyloidogenic protein, i.e., compounds capable of blocking the development of AA amyloidosis do not show in-vitro binding and/or anti-fibrillogenic activity against Aβ or IAPP fibril formation.[11]

One specific compound, 3-amino-1-propanesulfonic acid (3APS), has been identified as a potential therapeutic candidate and is undergoing clinical development. 3APS was found to bind preferentially to soluble Aβ, to maintain Aβ in a soluble form, and to reduce Aβ deposition in vivo.

3APS PREFERENTIALLY BINDS SOLUBLE Aβ

The ability of 3APS to bind Aβ was determined by electrospray mass spectrometry (Figure 4.1). 3APS was found to bind equally well to both $A\beta_{40}$ and $A\beta_{42}$, with more than 50% of the peptide bound to 3APS. The fact that the compound binds well to both Aβ peptides also indicates that this compound does not bind the carboxy-terminal region of the peptide, but most likely interacts in the central region of the peptide known to contain the GAG binding site. Additionally, 3APS does not bind fibrillar Aβ. Furthermore, 3APS was found not to bind to any of the major plasma proteins.

3APS REDUCES AMYLOID DEPOSITION IN VIVO

The TgCRND8 transgenic (tg) mouse model[14] was used to determine the ability of 3APS to interfere with the development of senile plaques. TgCRND8 hAPP mice express a double mutant (K760N/M671L and V717F) human βAPP695 (hAPP) transgene under the regulation of the Syrian hamster prion promoter (developed by the Centre for Research in Neurodegenerative Diseases, University of Toronto, ON, Canada). This hAPP mouse model is described as an early-onset model of brain amyloidosis, since thioflavine S

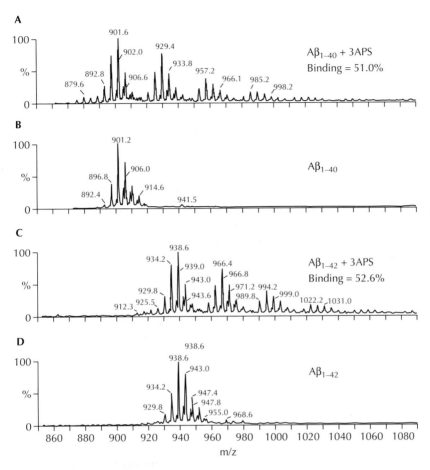

Figure 4.1

Binding of 3APS to $A\beta_{40}$ or $A\beta_{42}$ as determined by electrospray mass spectrometry. Solubilized $A\beta$ in water was mixed with 3 APS at a 1:10 ratio ($A\beta$:3APS). (A) $A\beta_{40}$ 20 μmol/L and 3APS 200 μmol/L; (B) $A\beta_{40}$ 20 μmol/L; (C) $A\beta_{42}$ 20 μmol/L and 3APS 200 μmol/L; (D) $A\beta_{42}$ 20 μmol/L. Only the +5 charged region of the spectrum is shown. Clusters result from a variable number of sodium ions associated with the corresponding species.

(ThioS)-positive brain amyloid deposits appear as early as 10 weeks of age. The total amount of brain amyloid in the TgCRND8 mice is greater than that seen in late-onset hAPP mice, such as the PDAPP mouse model. In the latter model, a 14-fold increase in total $A\beta$ brain concentration is seen between the ages of 12 and 18 months, where $A\beta$ reaches a concentration of 22 μg/g wet brain.[15] By comparison, TgCRND8 mice have been reported to have a 90-fold increase in their total $A\beta$ brain concentration between the ages of 10 and 25 weeks, to reach levels of ~31 μg/g wet brain.[16]

Adult TgCRND8 mice (9 ± 1-week-old) were given a single daily subcutaneous (sc) injection of 30 mg/kg or 100 mg/kg of 3APS for a period of 8 weeks (sc injections were used for convenience; oral administration of 3APS resulted in a brain pharmacokinetic profile similar to that seen with sc injections). At the termination of the treatment, mice were transcardially perfused, brains were excised, and the extent of cortical amyloid deposits was assessed by histochemistry following staining with ThioS. Stained sections were evaluated by image analysis (Image Pro Plus). To determine the number of plaques as well as the percent area of the analyzed region occupied by plaques, analysts were blinded to the identification of each treatment group.

Amyloid was not present at the initiation of the treatment of adult mice (baseline: 9-week-old). Adult mice treated with 100 mg/kg/day of 3APS for 8 weeks showed a significant reduction in amyloid deposition in the cortical brain region. As shown in Figure 4.2A, the number of plaques (i) and the percent cortical area occupied by plaques (ii) were significantly reduced by more than 30% ($p = 0.028$) in the animals treated with 100 mg/kg/day. Results obtained in the 30 mg/kg/day treatment group also showed an inhibitory effect on amyloid deposition that did not reach statistical significance but suggested a dose-dependent response to treatment. Figure 4.2B shows representative images of ThioS-stained sections of cortical regions of mice treated with the vehicle (i) or with 100 mg/kg/day of 3APS (i) or with the vehicle (ii) for 8 weeks; a marked decrease in the number and size of senile plaques is seen in the treated mice.

3APS was also found to have a profound dose-related effect on $A\beta$ plasma concentration, with a 37% and 61% reduction in $A\beta_{40}$ at 30 mg/kg/day and 100 mg/kg/day, respectively. $A\beta_{42}$ plasma levels were reduced by 31% and 66% in animals receiving 30 mg/kg/day and 100 mg/kg/day of 3APS, respectively (data not shown). TgCRND8 mice have 12 times more total $A\beta$ in their plasma than PDAPP mice (2000 ng/ml vs 160 ± 29 ng/ml).[17] The high $A\beta$ levels and the early onset, which characterize the TgCRND8 model used here, emphasize the significance of the 30% reduction obtained in such a short treatment duration.

The significant decrease in amyloid deposition and the substantial reduction in $A\beta_{40}$ and $A\beta_{42}$ plasma concentrations seen in treated adult animals led us to determine whether the soluble and insoluble fractions of $A\beta_{40}$ and $A\beta_{42}$ were both affected during treatment. To determine the level of brain $A\beta_{40}$ and $A\beta_{42}$ soluble and insoluble fractions, a second set of 9-week-old TgCRND8 animals were treated with 3APS for 9 weeks. Mice used for this experiment were the TgCRND8 N5 generation of a cross between B6 and FVB strains. This cross resulted in a greater total $A\beta$ plasma concentration (6000 ng/ml) than that found in the N2 generation, which was used in the first experiment (~2000 ng/ml). To maintain a 3APS:$A\beta$ ratio similar to that reached in the first experiment, mice were treated with 500 mg/kg/day of 3APS for 8 weeks (3APS pharmacokinetic profile shows linearity between 100 mg/kg and 500 mg/kg). Brain homogenates were evaluated for their soluble and insoluble $A\beta_{40}$ and $A\beta_{42}$ contents by ELISA. As seen in Figure 4.3, 3APS affected both soluble and

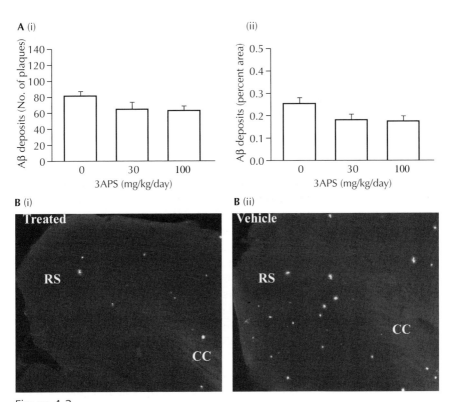

Figure 4.2

3APS treatment reduces murine cortical Aβ plaque formation. Mice were treated with 3APS for 8 weeks. Brain sections were stained with ThioS and amyloid burden was evaluated. (A) Effect of 3APS on the number of ThioS⁺ plaques per entire neo-cortical section (i) and percent of cortical surface area occupied by plaques (ii). (B) ThioS staining of representative histological brain sections of TgCRND8 mice following an 8-week treatment period with 100 mg/kg/day of 3APS (i) compared with non-treated mice (ii). RS: retrosplenial cortex; CC: corpus callosum.

insoluble Aβ fractions in the brain, reducing the soluble and insoluble fractions of both $A\beta_{40}$ and $A\beta_{42}$ by almost 40% and 25%, respectively. These results are consistent with the earlier findings using image analysis. 3APS was previously shown to cross the blood–brain barrier to exert its activity.[13] When both brain soluble $A\beta_{42}$ levels and 3APS brain concentration at steady state were compared, 3APS was found to be in a 24-fold excess compared to soluble $A\beta_{42}$ levels.

Preclinical toxicology studies showed that 3APS did not have any significant detrimental side effects when administered at high doses to dogs and rats (data not shown). This pharmacologic profile made 3APS an attractive anti-amyloid therapeutic candidate for AD. The ultimate proof-of-concept of the beneficial

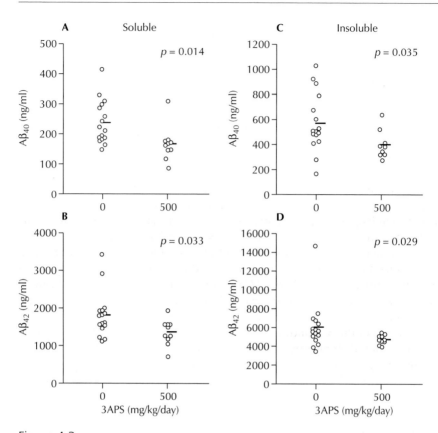

Figure 4.3

Effect of 3APS on the level of soluble and insoluble $A\beta_{40}$ and $A\beta_{42}$ in brain homogenates of animals treated for 9 weeks. Soluble $A\beta_{40}$ (A) and $A\beta_{42}$ (B) and insoluble $A\beta_{40}$ (C) and $A\beta_{42}$ (D) recovered from perfused brain homogenates of control (0 mg/kg/day) or treated animals (500 mg/kg/day 3APS) for 9 weeks. $A\beta$ levels were determined on brain homogenates by ELISA: 3APS did not interfere in the ELISA assay. Open circles represent values from individual animals; bars represent mean values. All values are expressed per gram of wet brain. Statistical analysis was done using the Mann–Whitney rank sum test.

effect of targeting the amyloid cascade remains the demonstration of clinical efficacy in patients with AD. Results obtained in a phase 2 clinical trial demonstrate that targeting soluble $A\beta$ with a new class of compounds represented by 3APS shows promise for the treatment of AD.

3APS IN PATIENTS WITH MILD-TO-MODERATE ALZHEIMER'S DISEASE

Phase 2 clinical study design

The phase 2 clinical study was designed to assess the safety, tolerability, and pharmacokinetic profile of 3APS in patients with mild-to-moderate AD (Mini-Mental State Examination (MMSE) 13–25). 3APS was administered to patients in a 3-month randomized, double-blind, placebo-controlled fashion. Groups of patients received 3APS orally at 50 mg, 100 mg, or 150 mg twice daily (bid). Patients were allowed to be on acetylcholinesterase inhibitor treatments. Those patients on symptomatic treatment had to be on stable therapy for at least 3 months prior to study entry. To better define and characterize the pharmacologic effects of 3APS, patients were evaluated for the presence of 3APS in cerebrospinal fluid (CSF), and its effect on $A\beta_{40}$ and $A\beta_{42}$ levels in the CSF and plasma. Patients were also evaluated for their cognitive function and global performance – ADAS-Cog (Alzheimer's Disease Assessment Scale – Cognitive), CDR-SB (Clinical Dementia Rating – Sum of the Boxes), and MMSE – at baseline and after 3 months of treatment.

At the end of the 3-month treatment period, all patients were offered entry into a 33-month-long open-label extension study. In this ongoing study, patients are given 150 mg 3APS bid. 3APS safety and efficacy continue to be investigated and patients are evaluated for their cognitive function and global performance.

Phase 3 study design

Results obtained in the phase 2 study have led to the initiation of a phase 3 study to investigate the safety and clinical efficacy of 3APS as a disease-modifying treatment in a multicenter, randomized, double-blind, placebo-controlled, and parallel-designed phase 3 study. This study is designed to enroll a total of 950 patients suffering from mild-to-moderate AD (MMSE 16–26). The patients are randomized into three groups to receive either placebo, 3APS 100 mg bid, or 3APS 150 mg bid for 18 months. Patients have to be on acetylcholinesterase inhibitor therapy with or without memantine therapy (NMDA receptor antagonist) for at least 4 months prior to study entry. The two primary endpoints to determine the clinical efficacy of 3APS consist of evaluating the change from baseline of cognitive functions and global performance as determined by ADAS-cog and CDR-SB scores following 18 months of treatment. Structural magnetic resonance imaging (MRI) will be used as a supportive evidence of disease-modifying treatment.

DISCUSSION

This chapter summarizes initial findings with 3APS, a novel low-MW anionic GAG mimetic. The results obtained in vitro and in vivo in TgCRND8 mice provide proof-of-concept that preferential binding to the soluble form of Aβ by a low-MW anionic compound effectively blocks the deposition of Aβ and favors its clearance from the brain. The effect is believed to be due mainly to the ability of compounds like 3APS to bind soluble Aβ and to disrupt Aβ protein–protein interactions, thereby reducing the potential of Aβ to organize as fibrillary senile plaques. 3APS also decreased brain and plasma soluble $Aβ_{40}$ and $Aβ_{42}$ concentrations, suggesting that it may affect the production or clearance of Aβ. We are now determining whether 3APS can also alter hAPP processing and/or Aβ clearance.

The two characteristic neuropathologic hallmarks of AD are the amyloid plaques and the neurofibrillary tangles (NFTs), which consist of intracellular inclusions of hyperphosphorylated tau. There is strong supporting evidence that the Aβ amyloidogenic process can be considered the triggering factor in the onset of AD and that tau hyperphosphorylation, NFT formation, and neuronal cell death are downstream consequences of Aβ fibrillogenesis.[16–19] 3APS intervenes early in the amyloid cascade, since it targets soluble rather than fibrillar Aβ. Clearance of Aβ by 3APS prior to its organization as fibrils could prevent and/or clear early tau pathology formation, as recently shown by Oddo et al[20] using Aβ immunotherapy. This finding supports the notion that by binding Aβ in its soluble form, 3APS could have an impact on the two neuropathologic lesions found in the brain of patients with AD. Acting early rather than late in the disease progression would also bring greater benefit to patients. Aβ amyloid deposits are also associated with the appearance of neuritic dystrophy, a chronic neuronal cell injury characterized by enlarged distorted axons and dendrites. Clearance of Aβ by immunotherapy was recently shown to lead to a rapid reversal of neuritic dystrophy.[21] The reduction of Aβ levels induced by 3APS prior to the organization of the amyloid protein in plaques may consequently induce the repair of damaged axons and dendrites and prevent any further damage caused by pre-deposited Aβ.

The compound's efficacy in reducing the amyloid burden in transgenic mouse brain led us to initiate the development of 3APS as a potential disease-modifying agent to stop the progression of AD in patients with mild-to-moderate AD. The phase 2 study was firstly designed to ensure the safety and tolerability of 3APS. In parallel, this phase 2 study allowed us to determine the pharmacokinetic profile of 3APS and its ability to penetrate the brain, as well as its pharmacologic effect on the amyloid protein in the CSF of patients. Results gathered during this phase 2 study showed that, as seen in animals, 3APS penetrates the brain and can reduce the level of amyloid protein in the CSF. The demonstration of the clinical efficacy of 3APS in patients with mild-to-moderate AD will be obtained in the phase 3 study. The study design will also allow us to determine whether an anti-amyloid approach targeting the soluble form of Aβ can lead to a disease-modifying treatment for AD.

ACKNOWLEDGMENTS

The transgenic human APP strain (TgCRND8) was obtained from the Centre for Research in Neurogenerative Disease, University of Toronto, ON, Canada. We wish to thank all those who have contributed to 3APS pharmacologic studies: J Paquette, C Morissette, P Krzykowski, M Yu, D Lacombe, A Aman, X Kong, and P Tremblay. We also wish to thank the Neurochem Drug Development team (R Poole, R Briand and J Laurin). Paul S Aisen, MD, is at the Department of Neurology of the Georgetown University Medical Center, Washington DC and Denis Garceau, PhD, is Senior Vice President at Neurochem, Laval, QC, Canada.

REFERENCES

1. McLean CA, Cherny RA, Fraser FW, et al. Soluble pool of Abeta amyloid as a determinant of severity of neurodegeneration in Alzheimer's disease. Ann Neurol 1999;46: 860–866.

2. Lue LF, Kuo YM, Roher AE, et al. Soluble amyloid beta peptide concentration as a predictor of synaptic change in Alzheimer's disease. Am J Pathol 1999;155:853–862.

3. McLaurin J, Yang D, Yip CM, Fraser PE. Review: modulating factors in amyloid-beta fibril formation. J Struct Biol 2000;130:259–270.

4. McLaurin J, Fraser PE. Effect of amino-acid substitutions on Alzheimer's amyloid-beta peptide-glycosaminoglycan interactions. Eur J Biochem 2000;267:6353–6361.

5. Sipe JD. Amyloidosis. Annu Rev Biochem 1992;61:947–975.

6. Verbeek MM, Otte-Holler I, van den Born J, et al. Agrin is a major heparan sulfate proteoglycan accumulating in Alzheimer's disease brain. Am J Pathol 1999;155:2115–2125.

7. Cotman SL, Halfter W, Cole GJ. Agrin binds to beta-amyloid (Abeta), accelerates Abeta fibril formation, and is localized to Abeta deposits in Alzheimer's disease brain. Mol Cell Neurosci 2000;15:183–198.

8. Gupta-Bansal R, Frederickson RC, Brunden KR. Proteoglycan-mediated inhibition of Abeta proteolysis: a potential cause of senile plaque accumulation. J Biol Chem 1995;270: 18666–18671.

9. Kisilevsky R, Fraser PE. Abeta amyloidogenesis: unique, or variation on a systemic theme? Crit Rev Biochem Mol Biol 1997;32:361–404.

10. Kisilevsky R, Lemieux LJ, Fraser PE, et al. Arresting amyloidosis in vivo using small-molecule anionic sulphonates or sulphates: implications for Alzheimer's disease. Nat Med 1995;1:143–148.

11. Gervais F, Morissette C, Kong X. Proteoglycans and amyloidogenic proteins in peripheral amyloidosis. Curr Med Chem (IEMA) 2003; 3:361–370.

12. Zhu H, Yu J, Kindy MS. Inhibition of amyloidosis using low-molecular-weight heparins. Mol Med 2001;7: 517–522.

13. Gervais F, Chalifour R, Garceau D, et al. Glycosaminoglycan mimetics: a therapeutic approach to cerebral amyloid angiopathy. Amyloid 2001; 8(Suppl 1):28–35.

14. Chishti MA, Yang DS, Janus C, et al. Early-onset amyloid deposition and cognitive deficits in transgenic mice expressing a double mutant form of amyloid precursor protein 695. J Biol Chem 2001;276:21562–21570.

15. Schenk D, Barbour R, Dunn W et al. Immunization with amyloid-beta attenuates Alzheimer-disease-like pathology in the PDAPP mouse. Nature 1999;400:173–177.

16. Hardy J, Selkoe DJ. The amyloid hypothesis of Alzheimer's disease: progress and problems on the road to therapeutics. Science 2002; 297: 353–356.

17. Lewis J, Dickson DW, Lin WL, et al. Enhanced neurofibrillary degenera- tion in transgenic mice expressing mutant tau and APP. Science 2001;293:1487–1491.

18. Gotz J, Chen F, van Dorpe J, et al. Formation of neurofibrillary tangles in P301l tau transgenic mice induced by Abeta 42 fibrils. Science 2001; 293:1491–1495.

19. Oddo S, Caccamo A, Shepherd JD, et al. Triple-transgenic model of Alzheimer's disease with plaques and tangles: intracellular Aβ and synaptic dysfunction. Neuron 2003;39: 409–421.

20. Oddo S, Billings L, Kesslak JP, et al. Aβ immunotherapy leads to clear- ance of early, but not late, hyper- phosphorylated tau aggregates via the proteasome. Neuron 2004;43: 321–332.

21. Brendza RP, Bacskai BJ, Cirrito JR, et al. Anti-Aβ antibody treatment pro- motes the rapid recovery of amyloid- associated neuritic dystrophy in PDAPP transgenic mice. J Clin Invest 2005:115:428–433.

5

Immunotherapy for Alzheimer's disease

David Wilkinson

INTRODUCTION

One of the most long-standing debates in Alzheimer's disease (AD) research concerns the relative importance, or the relative temporal relationships, of β-amyloid plaques and abnormally phosphorylated tau proteins, both of which are seen as histopathologic hallmarks of the disease. At present the pendulum has swung towards amyloid being the main protagonist. The amyloid cascade hypothesis states that overproduction, decreased clearance, or enhanced aggregation of the amyloid β-42 protein ($A\beta_{42}$) derived from an abnormal cleavage of the transmembranous amyloid precursor protein (APP) results in a cascade of events, culminating in cell death and dementia (Figure 5.1). A number of strategies are being explored as ways of preventing the oligomerization and aggregation of $A\beta_{42}$ or of increasing its removal from the CNS.

Attention has also been given to considering the process by which amyloid accumulation has its deleterious effects. One of these strategies has developed from the retrospective interpretation of a number of uncontrolled epidemiologic studies that suggest a protective effect of anti-inflammatory drugs. The belief that anti-inflammatory approaches would be the best way of treating, or of primary prevention of AD, was given weight by the finding that treatment with the NSAID (nonsteroidal anti-inflammatory drug) ibuprofen for 16 weeks reduced cortical plaque burden by 60% in one study of transgenic mice.[1] However, the early enthusiasm created from the epidemiologic data[2] has been undermined by the failure of a number of prospective studies using both non-selective and selective cyclooxygenase-2 (COX-2) inhibitors.[3] The hypothesis has not been satisfactorily disproved by these trials, as there is doubt that cyclooxygenases are involved in the selective reduction of $A\beta_{42}$.

It is also doubtful that they act through activating the peroxisome proliferator-activated receptor (PPAR)-γ, as the potent PPAR-γ agonist pioglitazone had a much more modest effect on reducing $A\beta_{42}$ levels in the same animal model. The effect of NSAIDs may be on γ-secretase, thus inhibiting production of $A\beta_{42}$ and increasing $A\beta_{38}$. Unfortunately, the NSAIDs used in the trials were not thought to have this effect; however, one drug, R-flurbiprofen, is currently being evaluated.

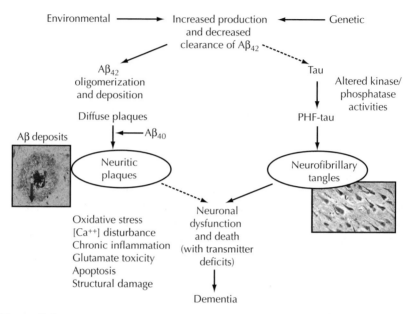

Figure 5.1
The amyloid cascade hypothesis

This failure of NSAID clinical trials has added strength to the view which argues that stimulating the natural inflammatory processes in the brain may be a better way of preventing deposition of, or the removal of, accumulations of unwanted proteins. Although to some a counterintuitive view this theory captured the imagination of the AD community, with huge interest in the first trials of the Elan (AN1792) vaccine in 2003. Unfortunately, an unexpected meningoencephalitis in 6% of subjects prevented the studies completing. Subsequently, a number of reports, many with a hint of schadenfreude, seemed to be writing off AD vaccines. However, these obituaries were a little premature, and a number of strategies are being developed to further explore this approach.

The immunotherapy approach relies heavily on our knowledge of microglia, which are the tissue macrophages of the central nervous system (CNS). Microglia associate with fibrillar Aβ, extending processes onto the plaque, where they undergo a phenotypic activation. Microglial activation is accompanied by a wide range of proinflammatory molecules that mediate the fulminating activation of these cells and the associated astrocytosis. Since activated microglia are seen in the earliest stages of any CNS disease, they are seen as a potential destructive force, promoting CNS inflammation. Consequently, many therapies for CNS neurodegenerative and inflammatory diseases have been directed at suppressing microglial function. Any inflammatory process can have both beneficial and malign effects; activation may be necessary to destroy unwanted pathogens or apoptotic cells, but if unprovoked it could have the potential to be toxic. There is evidence to suggest that microglia play an important role during the development and maintenance of CNS function that may go beyond simple defense against pathogens.[4] Molecular analysis of microglial phenotypes and function has shown that microglia are a unique CNS-specific type of tissue macrophage that are highly heterogeneous within the healthy CNS. They are not only exquisitely tailored to specific regions of the CNS but also to specific pathologic insults. Consequently, the wholesale suppression or activation of microglia is likely to be an ineffective strategy, with the potential to promote damaging outcomes.

The early attempts at vaccination may in retrospect appear to have lacked finesse, but they have given a unique opportunity to explore the relevance of amyloid to normal brain function and insight into whether strategies that remove it are harmful. Even if the removal of amyloid is not associated with improved function, it will still add to our understanding of the disease process.

ACTIVE IMMUNIZATION WITH AMYLOID B PEPTIDE IN PDAPP MICE

The first publication on a vaccination approach for AD was the paper from Schenk and the Elan Corporation, demonstrating the positive effects of vaccination in transgenic mice.[5] This landmark paper used the PDAPP transgenic mouse which overexpresses mutant human APP – in which the amino acid valine at position 717 is replaced by phenylalanine – and develops, very predictably by age and brain region, extracellular amyloid deposition resembling the plaques seen in AD as well as astrocytosis and neuritic dystrophy.

The researchers took the mice at 6 weeks, just prior to the development of plaques, and gave them monthly intraperitoneal injections of $A\beta_{42}$ until they were 13 months old. Dramatic histologic pictures showed that plaque deposition and the accompanying gliosis and neuritic dystrophy were prevented as compared with mice injected with PBS (adjuvant alone) or serum amyloid P protein, or controls left untreated (Figure 5.2).

The researchers then immunized mice from 11–18 months (an age at which they would have substantial plaque deposits) and showed in the $A\beta_{42}$-immunized mice that not only had the plaque density not increased but also that levels of cerebral $A\beta_{42}$ were lower than in 12-month-old untreated mice. The implication was that immunization not only prevented deposition but also caused removal of established plaques.

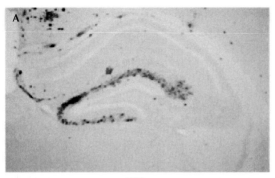

PBS

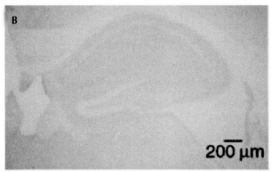

AN1792

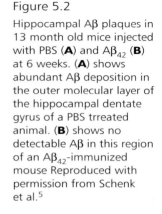

Figure 5.2

Hippocampal Aβ plaques in 13 month old mice injected with PBS (**A**) and Aβ$_{42}$ (**B**) at 6 weeks. (**A**) shows abundant Aβ deposition in the outer molecular layer of the hippocampal dentate gyrus of a PBS trreated animal. (**B**) shows no detectable Aβ in this region of an Aβ$_{42}$-immunized mouse Reproduced with permission from Schenk et al.[5]

BENEFITS OF ACTIVE IMMUNIZATION IN MICE

The beneficial effect of clearance of plaque from the mouse brain was provided by two further transgenic models. Janus et al,[6] using repeated intraperitoneal injections of Aβ$_{42}$ in the TgCRND8 mouse, showed that as well as decreased plaque burden (a 50% reduction in plaques but no reduction in total Aβ levels in the brain) the mice showed improved behavior in the Morris water maze, a commonly used test of reference memory. Morgan et al,[7] using two different transgenic mouse models and subcutaneous injections of Aβ$_{42}$, showed a partial reduction in plaques associated with improved performance in the radial-arm maze, a test of working memory. Later, these mice, at an age when they show memory deficits, were performing superiorly to control transgenic mice and at the same level as non-transgenic mice.

Neither of these mice models demonstrated the complete removal of Aβ$_{42}$, but by whatever mechanism – whether by partial clearance or modulation of some particularly toxic Aβ species is not clear – they seemed to show cognitive benefits.

PASSIVE IMMUNIZATION IN MICE

A similar but slightly less pronounced reduction in cerebral Aβ burden in PDAPP mice was obtained by weekly injections of a variety of monoclonal and polyclonal antibodies, although not all were effective.[8] In fact, only those recognizing the amino (N) terminus of $A\beta_{42}$ were able to prevent the formation of Aβ fibrils and invoke plaque clearance, and it was clear the entire 1–42 residues were not necessary. High affinity of the antibody for the Fc receptors on the microglia seemed more important than the affinity for Aβ itself, and complement activation was not necessary for plaque clearance. One hypothesis of how the beneficial effects of immunization are mediated is through the transport of anti-Aβ antibodies across the blood–brain barrier, where they bind to the Fc receptors on the microglia, inducing phagocytosis of the Aβ deposits in the brain.[9] Several authors have also shown substantial increases in plasma Aβ after passive immunization, suggesting an alternative method of plaque removal based on dialysis of soluble Aβ from brain to periphery, which is called the peripheral sink hypothesis. This has been supported by the finding that the monoclonal antibody 266, which does not bind to plaques, was still associated with amyloid reduction after passive administration.[10] Several studies have shown that immunization with a variety of antibodies to different epitopes of $A\beta_{42}$ can produce high antibody titers but only those to the N terminus, which bind to plaque in vitro, were associated with plaque clearance.[9] Antibody 266 is unique in its ability to reduce amyloid burden without binding to plaques and may be effective because of it unusually high affinity for soluble Aβ, producing a net flux of Aβ from the brain to the periphery, which over time would decrease the amyloid load.

Aβ IMMUNOTHERAPY AND TAU

One criticism of the transgenic mouse models used so far is that they do not adequately model AD, which is characterized by both Aβ plaques and neurofibrillary tangles. A study using a triple transgenic model (3xtg-AD) that develops both of the hallmark lesions in relevant brain regions showed that Aβ immunotherapy not only reduces extracellular Aβ plaques but also intracellular Aβ and most notably the clearance of early tau pathology.[11]

The researchers found that tau immunotherapy with the anti-tau monoclonal antibody HT7 had no discernible effect on tau pathology and no effect on amyloid pathology either. Interestingly, although the Aβ deposits were cleared within 3 days post-injection, the tau lesions were not reduced until 5 days. Aβ deposits returned by 30 days, but the tau pathology only returned to previous levels by day 45. The removal of tau was dependent on the proteasome, as blocking its function prevented the immunotherapy-mediated clearance. It was concluded that Aβ interferes with proteasome activity, so that immunotherapeutic removal of Aβ, by removing this interference, allowed the normal clearance of tau to take place. This would explain the delay in tau removal and its return not occurring until after Aβ returned, which also supports the amyloid cascade hypothesis. The clearance of tau also depended on the phosphorylation state, as late-stage hyperphosphorylated tau aggregates were unaffected by the Aβ antibody treatment.

These results suggest that Aβ immunotherapy may effectively clear Aβ and, provided that it is administered early in the disease course, tau pathology as well.

CLINICAL STUDIES

Phase 1b

The animal data and safety data in volunteers provided the rationale for studies in patients and the first dose-finding and immunogenicity study was started in April 2000 in the United Kingdom.[12] This was a phase 1b, randomized, double-blind, multiple-dose, dose escalation study conducted at four study sites and involved 80 patients with mild-to-moderate AD. Twenty patients were enrolled in each of four dose groups and randomly assigned to receive treatment in a 4:1, active:control ratio. In each dose group, treatment was administered as a 1 ml intradeltoid injection of 50 µg or 100 µg QS-21 (a surface-active saponin used as immunogenic adjuvant) alone or in combination with 50 µg or 225 µg AN-1792 (human aggregated $A\beta_{1-42}$) at Weeks 0, 4, 12, and 24.

After an interim data review to assess tolerability and immunogenicity, the study protocol was amended to add an optional extension phase (up to a total of 84 weeks after the first injection) that permitted patients to receive additional study injections at weeks 36, 48, 60 and 72. In the extension phase, the formulation of active and control immunizations was modified by the addition of 0.4% polysorbate 80 (PS-80) to improve product stability.

The primary objective of the study was safety and tolerability; the secondary objective of the study was to determine the immunogenicity of four dose combinations of AN1792 plus QS-21 in order to inform the protocol of a larger phase 2a study. Serology testing was performed using a reagent that could detect three kinds of immunoglobulins: IgG, IgM, and IgA. However, the reagent was not specific and, therefore, the anti-AN1792 titer detected in this study was classified simply as an Ig titer.

The study was not powered for efficacy, but four exploratory parameters were measured. Within each overall treatment group, the baseline characteristics were comparable among individual dose groups.

Donepezil HCl was the most frequently reported concomitant medication. All 80 patients received at least two injections of study treatment. A total of 73 (91.3%) patients received all four injections scheduled for the original protocol phase (59 AN1792 + QS-21 patients and 14 QS-21 patients). Of the

64 patients who entered the protocol extension phase, 57 (89.1%) received seven injections and 33 (51.6%) received all eight injections.

Responders were defined as patients with an antibody titer ≥1:1000 at 4 weeks after an injection and/or a titer ≥1:5000 at any time point after an injection.

Of the 51 AN1792-treated patients who entered the protocol extension, 29 (56.9%) were considered anti-AN1792 Ig antibody responders at some point during the study (Table 5.1).

A notable increase in the proportion of responders was observed after Injection 5 for all dose groups except AN1792 50 µg + QS-21 50 µg. A greater proportion of patients treated with the 225 µg dose of AN1792 were responders than those treated with the 50 µg dose of AN1792; therefore, AN1792 225 µg + QS-21 100 µg were chosen as the doses for the subsequent phase 2a study that started in October 2001.

There were 19 adverse events (AEs) reported as related to study treatment (18 active, 1 placebo): the most common were injection site pain, confusion, and hostility. There were 4 severe treatment-related AEs: worsening of dementia in a patient on placebo; and hostility, hallucinations, confusion, encephalitis in patients on AN1972. The patient with meningoencephalitis was only diagnosed at postmortem 1 year after withdrawal from the study with what was thought to be a primary CNS neoplasm.

Histopathologic findings

The postmortem findings in this patient were the first analysis of human neuropathology after immunization with AN1792 and, as such, are worth

Table 5.1	Anti-AN1792 antibody responders through week 84 (injections 1–8)[a]				
	Number of patients for AN1792 (QS-21)				
Injection	50 µg (50 µg) n = 10	50 µg (100 µg) n = 15	225 µg (50 µg) n = 15	225 µg (100 µg) n = 11	Total n = 51
1	0 (0.0)	0 (0.0)	0 (0.0)	0 (0.0)	0 (0.0)
2	0 (0.0)	0 (0.0)	1 (6.7)	0 (0.0)	1 (2.0)
3	2 (20.0)	2 (13.3)	4 (26.7)	0 (0.0)	8 (15.7)
4	2 (20.0)	2 (13.3)	5 (33.3)	2 (18.2)	11 (21.6)
5	0 (0.0)	5 (33.3)	8 (53.3)	3 (27.3)	16 (31.4)
6	2 (20.0)	5 (33.3)	9 (60.0)	4 (36.4)	20 (39.2)
7	2 (20.0)	6 (40.0)	10 (66.7)	6 (54.5)	24 (47.1)
8	2 (20.0)	7 (46.7)	9 (60.0)	5 (45.5)	23 (45.1)
Overall	2 (20.0)	7 (46.7)	13 (86.7)	7 (63.6)	29 (56.9)

[a] Antibody titers were measured before each injection.

considering.[13] She had four injections of AN1792 50 μg over 24 weeks with some suggestion of improvement, but 1 month after her fifth injection she rapidly declined. The diagnosis at that time was of an infiltrating primary brain tumor and, in accordance with the family's wishes, she was treated palliatively and died 1 year later after a pulmonary embolism. In comparison with 7 non-immunized cases, there were a number of unusual findings. Despite the presence of the diagnostic neuropathologic features of AD, there were extensive areas of neocortex that were entirely devoid of amyloid plaques (Figure 5.3). These areas contained tangles, neutropil threads, and cerebral amyloid angiopathy (CAA), as in the non-immunized cases, but lacked the plaque-associated dystrophic neurites (Figure 5.4). These areas also contained Aβ immunoreactivity associated with microglia. These findings strongly resembled the findings in the mouse models and suggested that the immune response had had similar effects in humans. There was also a T-lymphocyte meningoencephalitis and infiltration of the white matter with macrophages which appeared to be a side effect of immunization that had been seen in the subsequent phase 2a study. Similar findings were seen in a case from the phase 2a study who died after being diagnosed with meningoencephalitis following two injections of AN1792: T-lymphocytic infiltrate, focal depletion of diffuse and neuritic plaques, persistence of CAA, and collapsed plaques surrounded by active microglia.[14] A third case from a patient who did not have encephalitis has recently been published and shows similar, if slightly patchier, clear-

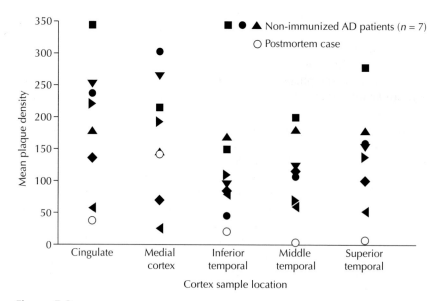

Figure 5.3

Reduced cortical plaque density compared with non-immunized Alzheimer disease patients. Reproduced with permission from Nicoll et al.[13]

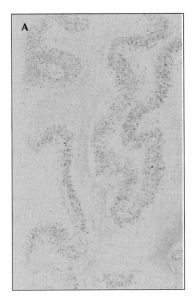
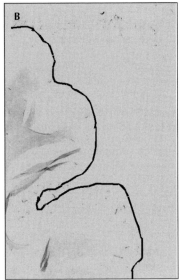

Figure 5.4
Apparent Aβ plaque removal in the temporal cortex. (**A**) Non-immunized
Alzheimer disease control. (**B**) Encephalitis case,

ance of amyloid, with only minimal T-cell infiltration or white matter involvement.[15] Again, there was no apparent reduction in the amyloid angiopathy or neurofibrillary tangles (Table 5.2).

Following our first case report[13] it was argued that any brain inflammatory process can cause the phagocytosis of amyloid,[16] as is the case after hemorrhagic stroke for instance.[13,16,17] However, in our case, the clearance was widespread and uniform, not patchy, and there were no hemosiderin deposits indicating any previous hemorrhagic lesions. Both microglial activation and T-cell infiltration can cause an acute picture that might be called encephalitis, and clearly it is important to know which is responsible. T lymphocytes, themselves, are unlikely to be involved in Aβ removal, whereas microglia are, and hence the next generation of immunotherapeutics are being designed to avoid the T-cell reaction, assuming that is the cause. If it is the microglial response that is responsible for the inflammatory process, it will be important to know. However, the appearances in subsequent cases and the findings of Aβ clearance in the absence of T-cell infiltration seem to argue for the encephalitis being a separate process from the Aβ removal and also that this is a specific effect of immunization.

From the phase 1b study, a further case of a patient who died from a cardiac aneurysm after only 4 months of immunotherapy has also been reported (Nicoll, pers comm). This patient also showed no evidence of

Table 5.2   Summary of neuropathologic findings

Phase 1b study: encephalitis case[13]
- T-lymphocytic infiltrate: CD4+
- Extensive areas of neocortex with few plaques
- Persistence of neurofibrillary tangles, neuropil threads, and cerebral amyloid angiopathy (CAA)
- Aβ immunoreactivity associated with microglia
- Macrophage infiltration of cerebral white matter

Phase 2a study: encephalitis case[14]
- T-lymphocytic infiltrate: CD4+, CD8+, CD3+, CD5+, CD7+
- Focal depletion of diffuse and neuritic plaques
- Persistence of CAA
- Collapsed plaques surrounded by active microglia

Phase 2a study: non-encephalitis case[15]
- Absence of white matter changes and minimal lymphocytic infiltrate
- Focal depletion of diffuse and neuritic plaques
- Persistence of neurofibrillary tangles and neuropil threads
- Aβ immunoreactivity associated with microglia/macrophages

meningoencephalitis and yet had signs of active phagocytosis of Aβ, as the considerable number of plaques that were still present were surrounded by abundant microglia containing amyloid. The inference drawn could be that amyloid removal was occurring, but that the patient had died before it had reached the level found in the other cases.

It is interesting to speculate on why the clearance of amyloid may have had no effect on the neurofibrillary tangles. It may be that there had not been sufficient time for the removal of tau following the plaque clearance, or more likely, as these patients died many months after their last injections, that, as in the 3xtg-AD mice, the hyperphosphorylated tangles were unaffected by the disinhibition of proteasome activity resulting from the removal of amyloid.

Phase 2a

The phase 2a study raised a number of further issues. In this multicenter safety and pilot efficacy study, 372 patients with mild-to-moderate AD were randomized to receive monthly injections of AN1792 225 μg + QS-21 100 μg or QS-21 100 μg alone. Dosing was discontinued after 4 reports of meningoencephalitis but follow-up continued and eventually 18 of 298 (6%) patients treated with AN1792 compared with 0 out of 74 on placebo were diagnosed.[18] There was no obvious relationship to the number of injections, with 16/18 occurring after the second injection, one case (the most severely affected patient) after the first injection, and one case (who initially had a favourable outcome) after the third injection. This was the patient described above who died with no evidence of encephalitis at postmortem.

Interestingly, there was no consistent correlation between the occurrence of meningoencephalitis and antibody titers, which were undetectable in three cases. Most cases occurred within 3 months of the first injection and none after 6 months, unlike the case in the phase 1b study. Twelve patients recovered within weeks, whereas 6 patients remained with disabling sequelae, 1 of whom died suddenly of inhalation several months after the encephalitis. Although it was clear that the immunization was associated with the meningoencephalitis, whether it was due to the T-cell response or whether it was due to microglial activation was unclear. Although modest, the efficacy outcomes were also interesting. An analysis of cognitive outcomes – including ADAS-cog (Alzheimer's Disease Assessment Scale – Cognitive), MMSE (Mini-Mental State Examination) and executive function – at 12 months in the 59 patients who had demonstrated an antibody response of any size, when compared to patients on placebo, showed no significant differences. Only one subset of the Wechsler Scale, the verbal delayed recall test, was significant with some trends in others. When the antibody responses were broken down into low and high, there seemed to be a slower rate of decline in the low-titer group and slight improvement in the high-titer group as compared with those patients with no response and those on placebo. There was also a reduction in CSF tau in those with an antibody response but no difference in $A\beta$ levels.

In a small subset of patients from one center in this study, a difference in cognitive response appeared to be correlated to the ability of antibody produced to bind to amyloid plaques. In this cohort, 20 of the 30 patients immunized developed antibodies against $A\beta$, as determined by a tissue amyloid plaque immunoreactivity (TAPIR) assay. This assay was statistically correlated with ELISA titers, but predicted therapeutic outcome more successfully. The differences between TAPIR and ELISA scores may reflect differences in epitope recognition and affinity of the binding reaction with $A\beta$ plaques, which may indicate the need to select therapeutically relevant epitopes within the $A\beta_{42}$ for future development of immunotherapy.[19]

The final twist in this study was demonstrated by the MRI (magnetic resonance imaging) scan results. It had been planned to make brain volumetric measurements at baseline, 12 months, and 15 months. After the dosing was stopped, the final scan was dropped, but the data from the 288 patients who had paired scans included 45 responders and 57 on placebo. The scans were rated blind, and it was found that the responders had a greater loss of brain volume than the controls. What is more, there was a direct correlation with antibody titer. Patients who had higher titers showed greater loss of whole brain and hippocampal volume. Ventricular enlargement was also greater in patients with higher titers, all measures being highly significant except the hippocampal volume. Some patients lost as much as 60 ml of brain volume considerably, which was more than the expected loss of around 5 ml per year in AD patients (which was the finding in the control group). Overall, patients with higher titers had a better outcome and also the largest drop in CSF tau. These apparently beneficial effects were achieved despite the greater loss of brain volume and greater ventricular enlargement normally regarded as indicative of atrophy associated with progression of the disease.

The patients from this Swiss cohort[19] also had a scan after 2 years and were found to have a slight recovery in their loss of whole brain volume, although the increase in volume of 2.8% in this small group (n = 11) is at the margins of the normal variation of this measurement and the comparison group of 3 patients without antibody response were not matched at baseline. This might indicate the return of amyloid, although the degree of volume loss would seem to be much greater than could be explained by removal of amyloid alone. Further autopsy cases may elucidate this point.

Conclusions from the clinical studies

A number of conclusions can be drawn from the two clinical studies and the resulting autopsies. Immunization with AN1792 + QS-21 elicited a positive antibody response to $A\beta_{42}$ in more than 50% of an elderly study population, with histopathologic findings strikingly similar to those seen in PDAPP mice (see Table 5.2). In the phase 1b study, patients on active treatment showed significantly less decline on the disability assessment for dementia (DAD) at week 84 than placebo patients, although no difference on cognitive scales Figure 5.5. In the phase 2a study, patients with higher antibody responses appeared to show advantage on cognitive outcomes, although with an increased brain volume loss at 1 year, than placebo patients. However, immunization with human aggregated $A\beta_{42}$ appears to trigger a sterile meningo-encephalitis in some patients, unrelated to their antibody response.

FURTHER STRATEGIES

Approaches other than immunization with the whole $A\beta_{42}$ peptide have been explored (Figure 5.6). As mentioned earlier, the capture of soluble Aβ by antibody 266, a high-affinity capture antibody, can reduce plaque by the peripheral sink mechanism. Antibodies against epitopes near the amino (N) terminus (Aβ1–5, Aβ1–10, Aβ3–5, Aβ5–11) bind with $A\beta_{42}$ and clear amyloid in vivo.[9,20] These epitopes are not the same ones associated with the T-cell response, which are from the mid region or carboxy (C) terminus. This may allow the development of N-terminus peptide conjugates, which may avoid the development of encephalitis.[9] It is also possible to use passive immunization with monoclonal antibodies to the same epitopes of $A\beta_{42}$ that bind to plaques and trigger Fc-mediated clearance. IgG2a antibodies have the greatest affinity for the phagocytic Fc receptors and provide the highest level of clearance. Plaque clearance seems independent of complement activation, as IgG1 antibodies, which cannot fix complement, were as effective as IgG2b, which can. Complement involvement in plaque clearance is likely to be more pronounced at higher doses of antibody, which would increase the density of

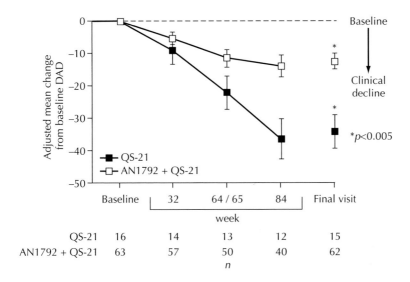

Figure 5.5
AN1792 slowed decline in disability assessment for dementia (DAD).

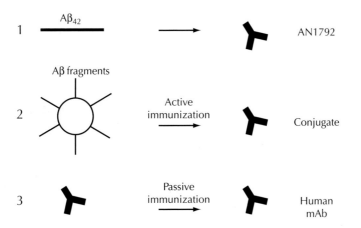

Figure 5.6
Amyloid beta (Aβ) immunotherapy approaches; mAb = monoclonal antibody.

antibody bound to plaques. It has been shown that activation of phagocytic cells through Fc receptors results in production of the anti-inflammatory cytokine interleukin (IL)-10 and the inhibition of the proinflammatory IL-12. Antibodies against Aβ may therefore resolve the chronic inflammatory response associated with Aβ plaques by clearing Aβ and through an anti-inflammatory cytokine response. This possibility has been tested in a very small pilot study in 5 patients using passive immunization with intravenous IgG prepared from plasma pools of donors.[21] IgG is used in other chronic neurologic conditions such as chronic inflammatory demyelinating polyneuropathy and it has been shown that human IgG contains antibodies to Aβ. The patients in this study had intravenous IgG over 6 months and showed a 30% reduction in cerebrospinal fluid (CSF) Aβ and an increase of 233% in serum Aβ but no change in $Aβ_{42}$ levels in either compartment. There was an associated increase in cognitive scores. The lack of change in $Aβ_{42}$ may suggest no alteration in plaque density, and the beneficial effects could be related to altered cytokine production by microglial cells via Fc receptors. Nasal vaccination with beta-amyloid peptide has also been explored in transgenic mice, as have oral vaccines, but as yet these have not been tested in humans.[22]

CONCLUSIONS

Immunotherapy is a fascinating approach to the treatment of AD. Although the initial Elan/Wyeth studies of AN1792 had to be halted, they provided a proof-of-concept, with enough encouragement from the outcome measures to further the research into safer conjugated vaccines and monoclonal antobodies. Elan has a passive immunization program with a monoclonal antibody already in clinical trials, and results are awaited with interest. The immunization approach has concentrated resources on the amyloid cascade as the main cause of AD. The findings in the postmortem studies of persistent CAA also favor amyloid as the core problem in the development of dementia. Aβ is normally eliminated from the brain, along with extracellular fluid, by bulk flow along the perivascular pathway. Age-related fibrosis of cerebral cortical and meningeal arteries leads to impaired drainage of Aβ along the perivascular pathway and, together with the production of Aβ by smooth muscle cells and perivascular cells, is responsible for accumulation of Aβ as CAA. Reduced elimination leads to increased concentration of soluble Aβ in the extracellular fluid of the brain parenchyma, and the increased concentration of soluble Aβ leads to the formation of insoluble Aβ plaques.[23] The failure of normal clearance mechanisms seems to be fundamental to the accumulation of Aβ, which in turn may inhibit the clearance of tau. Should a safe and effective immunization strategy be developed it would clearly be most beneficial in the early stages, where it would have most effect before significant plaque deposition had already resulted in abnormal axonal regeneration pathology. The increased loss of brain volume associated with the high antibody titers in the phase 2a study is of concern, but further animal studies may help to explain whether it is through loss of amyloid, astrocytes, or some other cause. If amyloid imaging can be used quantitatively, this may also help in future studies.

REFERENCES

1. Yan Q, Zhang J, Liu H, et al Anti-inflammatory drug therapy alters β-amyloid processing and deposition in an animal model of Alzheimer's disease. J Neurosci 2003;23(20):7504–7509.

2. Etminan M, Gill S, Samii A. Effect of nonsteroidal anti-inflammatory drugs and the risk of Alzheimer's disease: systemic review and review of observational studies. BMJ 2003;327:128–132.

3. Aisen PS, Schafer KA, Grundman, et al. Effects of refecoxib or naproxen vs placebo on Alzheimer's disease progression. JAMA 2003;289:2819–2826.

4. Carson M, Thrash CJ, Lo D. Analysis of microglial gene expression: identifying targets for CNS neurodegenerative and autoimmune disease. Am J Pharmacogenomics 2004;4(5):321–330.

5. Schenk D, Barbour R, Dunn W, et al. Immunization with amyloid-beta attenuates Alzheimer-disease-like pathology in the PDAPP mouse. Nature 1999;400:173–177.

6. Janus C, Pearson J, McLauren J, et al. Aβ peptide immunization reduces behavioural impairment and plaques in a model of Alzheimer's disease. Nature 2000;408:979–982.

7. Morgan D, Diamond DM, Gottschall PE, et al. Aβ peptide vaccination prevents memory loss in an animal model of Alzheimer disease. Nature 2000;408:982–985.

8. Bard F, Cannon C, Barbour R, et al. Peripherally administered antibodies against amyloid beta-peptide enter the central nervous system and reduce pathology in a mouse model of Alzheimer's disease. Nat Med 2000;6:916–919.

9. Bard F, Barbour R, Cannon C, et al. Epitope and isotype specificities of antibodies to β-amyloid peptide for protection against Alzheimer's disease-like neuropathology. Proc Natl Acad Sci USA 2003;100:2023–2028.

10. Citron M. Strategies for disease modification in Alzheimer's disease. Nature Rev Neurosci 2004;5:677–685.

11. Oddo S, Billings L, Kesslak JP, et al. Aβ immunotherapy leads to clearance of early, but not late, hyperphosphorylated tau aggregates via the proteasome. Neuron 2004;43:321–332.

12. Bayer AJ, Bullock R, Jones RW, et al. Evaluation of the safety and immunogenicity of synthetic Aβ42 (AN1792) in patients with Alzheimer's disease. Neurology 2005;64:94–100.

13. Nicoll J, Wilkinson D, Holmes C, et al. Neuropathology of human Alzheimer's disease following immunization with amyloid β-peptide: a case report. Nat Med 2003;9(4):448–452.

14. Ferrer I, Boada Rovira M, Sanchez Guerra M, et al. Neuropathology and pathogenesis of encephalitis following amyloid-beta immunization in Alzheimer's disease. Brain Pathol 2004;14(1):11–20.

15. Masliah E, Hansen L, Adame A, et al. Abeta vaccination effects on plaque pathology in the absence of encephalitis in Alzheimer's disease. Neurology 2005;64:129–131.

16. Akiyama H, McGeer P. Specificity of mechanisms for plaque removal after A beta immunotherapy for Alzheimer disease. Nat Med 2004;10:117–118.

17. Nicoll JA, Wilkinson D, Holmes C, et al. Specificity of mechanisms for plaque removal after Abeta immunotherapy for Alzheimer disease. Nat Med 2004;10:118–119.

18. Orgogozo J-M, Gilman S, Dartigues J-F, et al. Subacute meningoencephalitis in a subset of patients with AD

after Aβ42 immunization. Neurology 2003;61:46–54.

19. Hock C, Konietzko U, Streffer JR, et al. Antibodies against beta-amyloid slow cognitive decline in Alzheimer's disease. Neuron 2003;38:547–554.

20. McLaurin J, Cecal R, Kierstead ME, et al. Therapeutically effective antibodies against amyloid-beta peptide target amyloid-beta residues 4-10 and inhibit cytotoxicity and fibrillogenesis. Nat Med 2002; 8:1263–1269.

21. Dodel RC, Du Y, Depboylu C, et al. Intravenous immunoglobulins containing antibodies against β-amyloid for the treatment of Alzheimer's disease. J Neurol Neurosurg Psychiatry 2004;75:1472–1474.

22. Lemere CA, Maron R, Selkoe DJ, et al. Nasal vaccination with beta-amyloid peptide for the treatment of Alzheimer's disease. DNA Cell Biol 2001;20:705–711.

23. Nicoll JA, Yamada M, Frackowiak J, et al. Cerebral amyloid angiopathy plays a direct role in the pathogenesis of Alzheimer's disease. Pro-CAA position statement. Neurobiol Aging 2004;25:589–597.

6
Cholesterol, copper, and statin therapy in Alzheimer's disease

D Larry Sparks, Suzana Petanceska, Marwan Sabbagh, Donald Connor, Holly Soares, Charles Adler, Jean Lopez, Nina Silverberg, Kathryn Davis, Suhair Stipho-Majeed, Sherry Johnson-Traver, Paul Volodarsky, Chuck Ziolkowski, Jeff Lochhead, Patrick Browne

INTRODUCTION

Investigation of a possible role for cholesterol in Alzheimer's disease (AD) was a solitary endeavor during the late 1980s and most of the 1990s. The initial data linking AD neuropathology with coronary artery disease (CAD) and cholesterol among the non-demented met with significant resistance, requiring nearly 4 years for publication.[1]

These findings prompted studies identifying AD-like amyloid beta (Aβ) immunoreactivity in the brains of cholesterol-fed rabbits as the best small animal model of human CAD.[2] This resulted in formulation of the hypothesis that chronically increased circulating cholesterol leads to increased central cholesterol and accumulations of Aβ.[3,4] In the first study assessing a possible mechanism, Bodovitz and Klein showed in 1996 that cholesterol caused a shift of amyloid precursor protein (APP) metabolism from alpha to beta products in cultured cells.[5] In the following years, multiple groups reported that dietary cholesterol increased Aβ pathology in a variety of mouse models of AD, and that lowering cholesterol levels reduced Aβ production. In 1999, the first double-blind, randomized placebo-controlled clinical trial testing the possible benefit of a cholesterol-lowering statin (atorvastatin) in the treatment of AD (Alzheimer's Disease Cholesterol-Lowering Treatment trial; ADCLT) was funded, and the initial report of epidemiologic data suggested that prior use of cholesterol-lowering statins may be associated with a reduced risk of AD later in life. The ADCLT initiated recruitment in 2000 and, since then, there has been an explosion in the number of studies investigating the link between cholesterol and AD. This includes eight epidemiologic studies investigating statin use and risk of AD, six short-duration randomized or open-label statin clinical trials in AD patients, and six AD-related clinical trials of statins in non-demented patients, in addition to 20 review articles on the subject.[6–15] A number of these reviewers suggest that cholesterol and statins have drawn sufficient attention to warrant clinical trials to test for clinical benefit in AD[16–18] and mild cognitive impairment (MCI).[19]

SUB-ANALYSIS OF THE ALZHEIMER'S DISEASE CHOLESTEROL-LOWERING TRIAL

Primary assessment of the clinical data obtained in the ADCLT was reported early in 2004.[20] We herein provide secondary assessment of data from the ADCLT (mild-to-moderate AD), report similar data from clinically evaluated individuals willing to donate their brain after demise (controls, MCI, and AD), and review the literature in relation to our current findings.

The data presented herein for the AD population are based on biochemical measures of blood samples and Mini-Mental State Examination (MMSE) scores obtained at the screening visit for individuals later randomized into the ADCLT and AD patients participating in the Brain Bank Program. Separate informed consent was sought and obtained from individuals participating in the Brain Bank Program at Sun Health Research Institute who obtain yearly clinical evaluation predicated on donation of their brain at demise. These individuals were evaluated clinically for cognitive function and establishment of a diagnosis of AD, MCI, or cognitively normal for attained age. A consensus diagnosis was required for those individuals deemed to be exhibiting MCI, employing the criteria of Petersen et al.[21,22] MCI is a stage of cognitive ability considered a forerunner to dementia.

Blood samples were collected for chemical assessment at the first clinical evaluation visit. In each individual (Brain Bank and ADCLT) we established circulating levels of cholesterol (total and HDL (high-density lipoprotein)), ceruloplasmin (copper chaperone[23]), and Aβ. Aβ levels were measured by ELISA, as described previously[24] for blood samples obtained at the initial clinical visit from Brain Bank subjects and at screen for ADCLT participants (presented cross-sectional data). Samples were run in multiple assays with a high assay-to-assay correlation (0.8–0.9). Aβ levels were measured using a two-step sandwich immunosorbent assay employing a DELFIA-based platform, as described previously[25] for screen and quarterly evaluation in the ADCLT (longitudinal data). Cross-sectional Aβ levels are express in fmol/ml and longitudinal Aβ levels are expressed in pg/ml. The correlation between cross-sectional data for screen values for ADCLT subjects and screen values for ADCLT participants in the longitudinal data for Aβ was $r^2 = 0.4$ ($p<0.01$).

The MMSE was administered as a measure of global function to evaluate disease progression in the ADCLT and the Brain Bank Program.[26] Rey's AVLT (Auditory Verbal Learning Test) was administered to each Brain Bank Program participant as part of their routine clinical evaluation of memory performance.[27] Executive function and visiospatial performance were measured using the Clock Draw Test[28] in Brain Bank Program participants. The capacity to identify differing odors by matching a particular aroma with a provided list of choices was assessed in Brain Bank Program participants using a smell identification test.[29]

Brain Bank control individuals were stratified according to performance on the MMSE and the Rey AVLT-A7 (Auditory Verbal Learning Test – delayed recall). The AVLT-A7 is a sensitive clinical instrument that assesses verbal memory. These controls were grouped based on their MMSE and the AVLT-A7 scores: high-function control group (MMSE = 30 and AVLT-A7 = 12–15), and a low-function control group (MMSE = 28–29 and AVLT-A7 = 5–11).[25]

Based on these clinically defined groupings of controls,[25] we discuss cross-sectional data from 42 controls (two groups), 21 MCI subjects, and 13 subjects with AD from the Brain Bank population. The MMSE, the Rey AVLT, and the Clock Draw Test were administered to each Brain Bank participant, and the University of Pittsburgh Smell Identification Test (UPSIT) was administered to a subset of these individuals. Screen values of MMSE scores, and cholesterol, ceruloplasmin, and Aβ levels are provided from 72 ADCLT individuals in this cross-sectional evaluation. Assessment of the AVLT-A7, Clock Draw Test, and UPSIT were not performed in the ADCLT. Data from a total of 148 individuals are presented: 18 high-function controls, 24 low-function controls, 21 MCI, and 85 AD (13 Brain Bank and 72 ADCLT) patients. We also discuss longitudinal data for the 63 ADCLT patients providing evaluable data (completing the first of four quarterly visits).

There was no difference in age or years of education between the control, MCI, and AD groups (Figure 6.1). Any Brain Bank subject with a diagnosis of a dementing disorder other than AD or taking a statin medication was excluded. Prior or ongoing statin use precluded participation in the ADCLT. This is important, as performance on the MMSE and AVLT instruments is education sensitive. A significant reduction in performance on the AVLT-A7, but not the MMSE, was detected in the MCI population (Figure 6.2). A significant reduction in ability on the MMSE and a further significant deterioration on the AVLT-A7 was identified among AD patients compared with subjects diagnosed MCI (see Figure 6.2). Consistent with these observations it was noted, while following changes in cerebrospinal fluid (CSF) Aβ levels in the transition from MCI to AD, that MCI patients converting to AD tended to have reduced delayed verbal recall at baseline.[30]

We found in a cross-sectional study of controls, MCI, and AD patients,[25] that scores on the Clock Draw Test, measuring executive function and visiospatial performance, was similar in both control groups, significantly reduced in the MCI population compared with controls, and not significantly different between the MCI and AD groups (see Figure 6.2). The AD patients had mild disease (mean MMSE score of 20), and had they been more severely affected the difference between MCI and AD may have been more pronounced and significant.

In these studies,[25] we also identified that the ability to discern differences on the UPSIT was similar for the control and MCI groups, but was significantly reduced in AD patients (see Figure 6.2). It has been suggested that this is merely a consequence of memory loss in the disorder, but it is of interest that

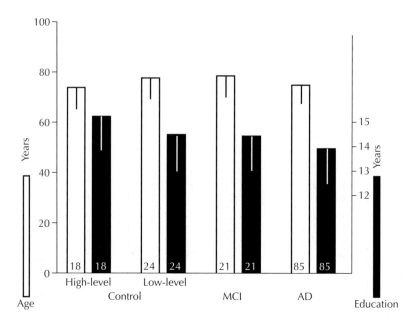

Figure 6.1

Age and education for the study groups. There was no difference in age and education in years for the Brain Bank populations of clinically evaluated individuals. There are two groupings of control: those with MCI and those with AD, including the age and education of AD patients (at screen) participating in the ADCLT.

this capability is retained among MCI patients showing significant deterioration in memory assessed by the AVLT-A7.

We also found[25] that circulating levels of $A\beta_{1-40}$ were significantly increased in the low-function control group compared with high-function controls, and that they were further significantly increased in MCI compared with low-function controls. In AD, the levels of $A\beta_{1-40}$ were not different from controls, but were on average significantly lower than levels among individuals with a diagnosis of MCI (Figure 6.3). Circulating levels of $A\beta_{1-42}$ did not vary significantly between the four groups, but were highest in the MCI group (not shown). These data for levels of $A\beta$ are for the most part consistent with previous reports. As we reported in plasma, one study indicates that decreased CSF $A\beta_{1-40}$ levels occur during the transition from MCI to AD.[30] Another study identified a decrease in CSF $A\beta_{1-40}$ in the transition from MCI to AD, but no change between control and MCI.[31] A third study suggested there are increased CSF $A\beta_{1-40}$ levels when comparing control with MCI.[32] More recently, a reduction in CSF $A\beta_{1-42}$ levels in the transition from MCI[24] to AD (35 mild, 26 severe) has been identified.[33]

A study investigating plasma, rather than CSF, identified no difference in $A\beta_{1-40}$ or $A\beta_{1-42}$ levels between controls, MCI, or AD.[34] Control individuals

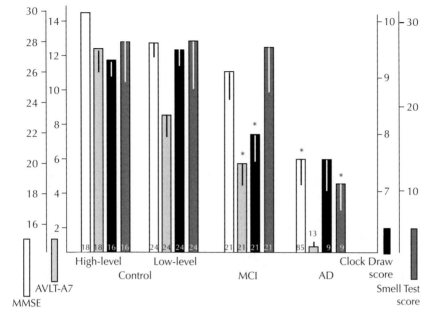

Figure 6.2

Mean group performance (± SEM) on the MMSE, AVLT-A7, Clock Draw Test, and UPSIT (smell identification test). The MMSE and AVLT-A7 were set by definition for the high- and low-function control groups. No difference on the Clock Draw Test or UPSIT was observed between the control groups. A significant deterioration on the MMSE and UPSIT was identified in AD compared with MCI and controls. Stepwise significant decreased performance on the AVLT-A7 occurred between control and MCI, and MCI and AD. A significant decreased score on the Clock Draw Test occurred between controls and MCI and AD, but was similar between MCI and AD.

were administered the CDR (Clinical Dementia Rating) and Blessed Dementia Scale, but were not stratified according to performance. A more recent study determined the plasma levels of only $A\beta_{1-42}$ in 88 MCI patients and 72 controls. No difference was seen between the two populations, but, when stratifying by sex, increased plasma $A\beta_{1-42}$ levels were identified in women with MCI and not men compared with controls.[35] Consistent with these observations, we found no difference in plasma $A\beta_{1-42}$ between the two control groups stratified according to clinical performance, MCI, and AD, although $A\beta_{1-42}$ levels tended to be higher in the MCI group compared with all other groups. We did not stratify the data according to sex of the participants, as noted above. Consistent with findings in CSF, we found that there were significant increases in plasma $A\beta_{1-40}$ between high- and low-function controls and again between low-function controls and individuals with MCI, which decreased to the levels observed in high-function controls among patients with AD (see Figure 6.3).

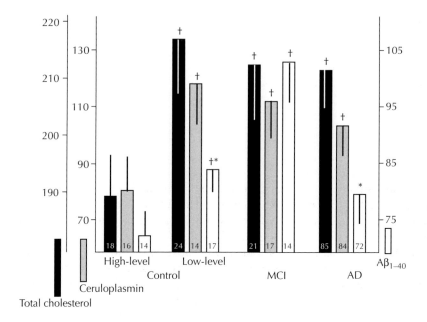

Figure 6.3

Mean group levels ($^+$ SEM) of circulating total cholesterol, ceruloplasmin, and $A\beta_{1-40}$ for Brain Bank control, MCI, and AD subjects, including screen values for AD patients participating in the ADCLT. Levels of total cholesterol and ceruloplasmin increased between high-function and low-function controls and remained elevated in MCI and AD. Levels of $A\beta_{1-40}$ increased between high-function and low-function controls and again between low-function controls and MCI; levels decreased in AD compared with MCI.

CHOLESTEROL IN ALZHEIMER'S DISEASE

Epidemiologic surveys suggest an association between risk of AD and presence of atherosclerotic heart disease,[36–41] as well as a link between a high fat/choles-terol diet and increased risk of AD.[42–45] Cholesterol levels are increased in the blood of AD patients,[42,46–49] and increased cholesterol has been observed in the AD brain as a function of ApoE allotype.[43,50] A half-dozen clinical studies suggest a link between cholesterol and AD:[50–56] one study reports a three-fold increased risk of AD with elevated serum cholesterol, even after adjusting for age and presence of the apolipoprotein E4 allele;[52] another study indicates that it is persistently elevated cholesterol levels in midlife that increases the risk of AD.[56] We have found that circulating total cholesterol levels are significantly increased in low-function controls compared with high-function controls (Figure 6.3).[25] Total cholesterol levels were similarly elevated in the low-function control, MCI, and AD populations compared with the high-function control population (Figure 6.3).[25]

Nevertheless, increased cholesterol synthesis in AD brain has not been reported; in fact, the level of mRNA for the rate-limiting enzyme in cholesterol synthesis (HMG CoA reductase) is unchanged in AD brain compared with age-matched controls,[57] which suggests a normal capacity to produce cholesterol and tends to support the premise that increased brain cholesterol promoting Aβ synthesis emanates from the blood.

Animal and culture studies

Initial studies in cholesterol-fed New Zealand White rabbits identified prominent neuronal accumulations of Aβ, as well as numerous other neuropathologic findings similar to features observed in AD brain.[58–63] Transgenic mouse models of AD have been shown to accumulate Aβ earlier or in greater abundance, or both, if administered excess cholesterol in the diet.[24,64–67] In the PS/APP mouse model of AD, dietary cholesterol has been shown to increase brain cholesterol and Aβ levels.[24] Mice with the APP695 Swedish mutation fed a high cholesterol diet experience increased brain Aβ, without an increase in brain cholesterol.[66] In the same mouse model, dietary cholesterol has been shown to increase both cholesterol and Aβ levels in the brain.[67] Likewise, mice with the APP v717f mutation fed a high fat/cholesterol diet exhibited elevated brain Aβ; this cholesterol-induced effect was more robust in males compared with females,[64] and was accelerated if apolipoprotein E was present.[65]

In-vitro studies have demonstrated that cholesterol is capable of shifting the metabolism of APP to production of amyloidogenic peptides.[68–73] It has generally been shown that cholesterol increases β-secretase and possibly γ-secretase activity to produce increased intracellular Aβ from newly synthesized APP.[68–74] The effect of cholesterol on APP metabolism is dose-related and not mediated via the low-density lipoprotein (LDL)-receptor.[68] Galbete et al showed that cholesterol causes a 60% decrease in APPs and a slight decrease in APP mRNA.[71] In contrast, a recent study[75] in transgenic mice suggested that a cholesterol diet enhances brain Aβ burden without a clear increase in brain cholesterol, and also reported that statins alter brain cholesterol distribution, indicating the medication may indirectly induce changes in Aβ, possibly by BBB (blood–brain barrier) interaction via nitric oxide (NO) and apolipoprotein E.[75]

Analogous cell culture studies have demonstrated that inhibition of the rate-limiting step of cholesterol synthesis with statin drugs reduces the level of Aβ produced.[69,70,72,76,77] In contrast, reducing cholesterol synthesis below a critical level can induce neuronal death.[78] The foregoing, coupled with evidence that Aβ can inhibit central cholesterol synthesis, provided the rationale for choosing atorvastatin (BBB impermeable) to test in the investigator-initiated ADCLT, and why it might be ill-advised to introduce a statin inhibiting central cholesterol synthesis in AD patients rampantly producing Aβ.[79]

Similar to culture studies, the BBB permeable cholesterol-lowering drug BM15766 administered to transgenic mice (PS1/APP) causes reduced levels of cholesterol and Aβ in the brain.[80] Similarly, simvastatin (BBB permeable) administered to guinea pigs maintained on a control diet reduced Aβ levels below those occurring naturally.[77] Administration of atorvastatin (BBB impermeable) to PS1/APP has been shown to reduce Aβ deposition in brain without reducing brain cholesterol levels.[81] A recent study provides contrasting evidence when testing the effect of the BBB-permeable lovastatin on brain Aβ levels in Tg2576 mice.[82] This statin reduced circulating cholesterol in both males and females, but caused an increase in Aβ in the brains of females but not males – without altering the levels of full-length APP, sAPPalpha (secreted APP after α-secretase metabolism), or presenilin 1 (PS1).[82] More recently,[83] studies tested the effect of lovastatin and pravastatin (BBB-impermeable statin) on Aβ and cytokine levels in 3-month-old TgCRND8 mice (mutant human APP) – after 1 month of treatment, both statins reduced total Aβ peptides and increased sAPPalpha, but only lovastatin increased tumor necrosis factor-alpha (TNFα) and interleukin 1-beta (IL-1β) and enhanced cerebral inflammation. This suggested that use of a BBB-impermeable statin may be safer in the treatment of AD,[83] a clear consideration in choosing atorvastatin for testing in the ADCLT.[79]

Other mechanisms for how cholesterol may promote Aβ production and accumulation and how statin therapy might elicit benefit in the treatment of AD are proposed. These include lipid-independent pleiotropic effects of statins.[84] One group of authors proposed that altered membrane transbilayer cholesterol distribution is the primary influence on Aβ production, rather than increased total cholesterol.[14] A number of investigators suggest that oxysterols and ester derivatives could mediate the effect of cholesterol's involvement in AD, suggesting genotypic differences in 24-hydroxylase, ACAT (acyl CoA: cholesterol acyltransferase), or ABC-A1 (cholesterol transport complex) as candidates for investigation.[11,85–87]

One group showed pravastatin pretreatment of human glioma cells reduced IL-6 and free radicals produced by $Aβ_{1-42}$ as an alternate mechanism by which statins may be of benefit in AD.[88] Another consideration in choosing atorvastatin for testing in the ADCLT was evidence that medication reduced circulating free radical markers and cholesterol in non-demented individuals, but atorvastatin produced no difference in circulating superoxide dismutase or glutathione peroxidase activity compared with placebo in the ADCL.[89]

Another hypothesis is that herpes simplex virus-1 (HSV-1) and *ApoE4* confer increased risk of AD, and statins could reduce the risk by reducing the spread of HSV-1 via lipid raft domain pathways.[90] Yet another group suggests statin therapy could be of benefit in AD by increasing apolipoprotein E levels, as there is gain of function during regeneration with increased levels of the lipoprotein.[9] This is probably not the case, as neither AD statin trial measuring apolipoprotein E content found increased levels. The study of simvastatin, lovastatin, and pravastatin identified decreased cholesterol, but no change in

circulating apolipoprotein E content with each statin.[91] In the ADCLT, atorvastatin significantly decreased circulating apolipoprotein E levels, starting at
3 months.[25] This is consistent with the previous suggestion that statin therapy
may be of benefit as a result of the reductions of apolipoprotein E levels produced.[92]

Statin medications induce modest increases in HDL-cholesterol among non-
demented individuals treated to reduce elevated cholesterol levels. Michikawa
proposed that the mechanism by which statins may produce benefit in AD is
by increasing HDL-cholesterol.[15] In contrast to this suggestion, data from the
ADCLT[25] indicate that, rather than increasing HDL-cholesterol, atorvastatin
initially produces no change and eventually significantly reduces HDL-cholesterol levels (Figure 6.4).

Most recently, Pedrini et al provided evidence that statins can stimulate the
non-amyloidogenic processing of APP as a result of inhibition of the iso-
prenoid branch of cholesterol synthesis, and that this mechanism involves the
Rho/Rho-kinase pathway,[93] suggesting a lipid-independent pleiotropic effect.
These authors also opined that the benefit of statin therapy in AD may be due
to reduced peripheral Aβ levels produced.[93] This is a controversial issue, as
there are conflicting clinical evidence. Controlled-release lovastatin reduces

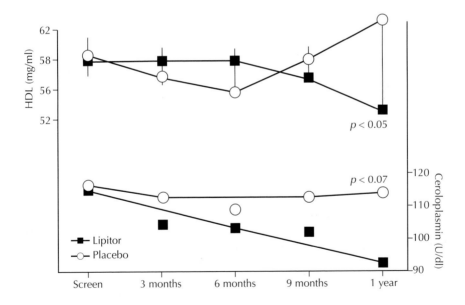

Figure 6.4

Normalized circulating HDL-cholesterol and ceruloplasmin levels at screen and all
visits for evaluable individuals (n = 63) participating in the ADCLT. The levels of
HDL-cholesterol were decreased in the atorvastatin group compared with placebo
at the 1-year time point only. A trend for a significant reduction in ceruloplasmin
levels occurred in the atorvastatin (Lipitor) group.

circulating Aβ levels in non-demented individuals,[94] and in a dose-related manner.[95] In contrast, no difference in circulating Aβ levels were observed when comparing non-demented individuals taking and not taking a statin.[96] In another study, non-demented subjects received either simvastatin or atorvastatin; both statins reduced circulating cholesterol but produced no change in circulating $A\beta_{1-40}$ or $A\beta_{1-42}$ levels.[97] Likewise, no change in circulating $A\beta_{1-40}$ or $A\beta_{1-42}$ levels were produced in non-demented hyperlipidemic patients administered pravastatin.[98]

In AD, reduced Aβ levels are noted in the CSF, but only in mildly affected patients treated with 80 mg of simvastatin/day.[99] Open-label treatment of AD patients with simvastatin (20 mg/day) for 12 weeks failed to alter Aβ levels in plasma.[100] Similarly, no reductions in circulating Aβ levels, but benefit on cognitive indices, were produced by atorvastatin in the ADCLT:[25] in fact, slight gradual increases in the circulating levels of both $A\beta_{1-40}$ and $A\beta_{1-42}$ were identified (Figure 6.5).

Epidemiologic studies

Since the initial epidemiologic investigation assessing the effect of statin use on later risk of AD, there have been 8 additional studies – most reporting

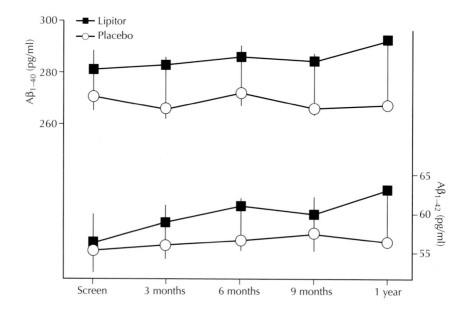

Figure 6.5

Mean plasma $A\beta_{1-40}$ and $A\beta_{1-42}$ levels at screen and all visits for all evaluable individuals ($n = 63$) participating in the ADCLT. Sight gradual increases observed in the atorvastatin (Lipitor) group compared with placebo were not significant.

some benefit with cholesterol-lowering therapy. Wolozin et al showed benefit associated with the use of lovastatin and pravastatin, but not simvastatin or non-statin therapy.[101] Jick et al showed benefit associated with cholesterol-lowering therapy, and not specifically with statin use.[102] At this point in time the Cache County data were assessed for reduced risk of AD associated with BBB-impermeable vs BBB-permeable statin use compared with non-statin users. The report of this first wave of assessment that suggested benefit of statin use, principally associated with those BBB-impermeable medications, met with clear opposition to publication.

Shortly thereafter, a study indicated that there was a significantly lower likelihood of prescribing statins to demented individuals.[103] The same year, Yaffe et al reported a modest reduction in the risk of AD associated with statin use in a study of women,[104] and Rockwood et al[105] provided evidence of a possible association between statin use and reduced risk of AD. A second assessment wave of the Cache County data indicated a less than significant reduction in the risk of AD with statin use, but suggested more promise among individuals treated with a BBB-impermeable statin; publication of this data continued to encounter opposition.

More recently, Zamrini et al reported the results of a nested case-control study of newly diagnosed AD ($n = 309$) and non-AD controls ($n = 3088$), assessing odds ratios (ORs) between AD and statin use. They identified a 39% reduced risk of AD in statin users compared with non-statin users (OR 0.61, 95% CI 0.42–0.87).[106] A retrospective cohort study of intelligence and cognition assessed at a young age and again in the 1980s indicated there were detrimental effects of neuroactive drugs and polypharmacy, but a significant beneficial effect with statin use.[107] A very recent epidemiologic study[108] identified no association between statin use and a reduced incidence of probable AD using a time-dependent proportional hazards statistical assessment model, but if analyzed as a case-controlled study a false-positive protective effect was obtained, suggesting that the statistics may have been inappropriate in previous studies that showed a positive effect. Similarly, the finally published form of the Cache County data indicated that there was no significant reduction in the risk of AD with statin use, but allowed for the possibility that some benefit could be provided with longer-term statin therapy.[109]

Clinical trials

While the ADCLT was ongoing, a number of investigators initiated studies testing a variety of statins for their effect on Aβ metabolism in both AD patients[91,99,100,110,111] and non-demented individuals,[94–97] and one study assessed cognitive performance in non-demented individuals in relation to statin use and observable changes in MRI scans.[112] Only the Simons et al 2002 study[99] and the ADCLT included a sufficient number of participants treated with a single statin to assess the therapy for any clinically identifiable beneficial effect on cognition.

The design of the ADCLT has been detailed previously.[3,4,113] Briefly, 72 mild-to-moderately affected AD patients were eligible to be randomized to either placebo or 80 mg/day of atorvastatin for a 1-year period. Sixty-seven participants received study medication, but only 63 individuals completed the first quarterly visit (13 weeks) and provided evaluable data (32 atorvastatin, 31 placebo). We evaluated change in performance on the MMSE,[26] ADAS-cog (Alzheimer's Disease Assessment Scale – Cognitive),[114] NPI (Neuropsychiatric Inventory),[115] CGIC (Clinical Global Impression of Change Scale),[116] ADCS-ADL (Alzheimer's Disease Cooperative Study – Activities of Daily Living),[117,118] and the GDS (Geriatric Depression Scale),[119] during the trial, and collected blood to assess change in cholesterol and Aβ levels produced. We have reported the initial clinical results of the ADCLT, where atorvastatin treatment, in the setting of continued cholinesterase inhibitor use, provided significant benefit on the ADAS-cog at 6 months ($p = 0.003$) and marginally significant benefit at 1 year ($p = 0.055$), while providing a trend for benefit on the CGIC and NPI and actual improvement on the GDS ($p < 0.04$) after 1 year of therapy.[89,113] The observed benefit on the MMSE produced by atorvastatin treatment did not reach significance at any time point, and there was no significant change identified on the ADCS-ADL. As expected atorvastatin treatment significantly reduced total, LDL, and VLDL (very low density lipoprotein) cholesterol levels.

As part of the rationale for the ADCLT, a mechanism was suggested that cholesterol coming from the blood in the wrong form (free) and in the wrong compartment (extraneuronal) influenced APP metabolism. Cholesterol is produced in ample quantities within brain cells and packaged for appropriate use therein (i.e. rafts). After synthesis, APP is transported by vesicle to the membrane for incorporation, such that the eventual extracellular N-terminal end of APP is protected inside the vesicle and the intracellular C-terminal end of APP remains in the intracellular milieu. This allows for appropriate orientation of APP upon 'docking' of the vesicle with the membrane. Because β-secretase has been shown to reside inside APP-containing vesicles, coupled with evidence that excess free cholesterol stagnates vesicle transport, reduced vesicle motility would promote β cleavage of APP within the vesicle. As noted above, cholesterol exerts its effect on the metabolism of newly synthesized, perhaps vesicularized APP. It is also proposed that excess free cholesterol could inhibit α-secretase metabolism of APP already inserted into the membrane, thus acting in the wrong form and in the wrong compartment.

As part of this mechanism it was proposed that cholesterol produced sufficient Aβ so as to overwhelm clearance pathways, culminating in central accumulation of the toxin. In addition, or alternately, this excess cholesterol could also exert direct effects on the cerebrovasculature or Aβ efflux to attenuate clearance and promote accumulation.

A significant problem arose as we embarked on the statin studies in humans. The ADCLT was based on data from the cholesterol-fed rabbit model of AD, and, as the ADCLT started, we found that dietary cholesterol no longer caused the accumulation of Aβ in the rabbit brain. In this same time frame, we finally became USDA (United States Department of Agriculture) accredited and initiated rabbit studies 'in house'. As we later discerned, the cholesterol-fed rabbits not exhibiting accumulations of Aβ were being administered distilled drinking water rather that local tap water as had been routine in past experiments. It was eventually disclosed that it was copper ion in the tap water that promoted the accumulation of Aβ. Cholesterol continued to cause the overproduction of Aβ but was cleared to the blood, where levels were increased, among animals maintained on distilled drinking water.[120] In animals fed dietary cholesterol and administered distilled drinking water with copper ion added (0.12 ppm), Aβ accumulated in the brain, and levels were only slightly increased in the blood. This clearly suggested that much of the Aβ in blood was produced in the brain and that copper ion introduced via the drinking water inhibited Aβ clearance from the brain.[120,121] This is consistent with findings in mouse models of AD, where the equilibrium of Aβ between brain and blood may vary with the level of its deposition in the brain.[122,123]

Significant memory deficits were observed in the cholesterol-fed rabbits on copper-supplemented distilled water, with central Aβ accumulations, compared with cholesterol-fed rabbits on unaltered distilled water, where there were increases of Aβ in the blood and not the brain.[121] Over 95% of the copper in human blood is transported by ceruloplasmin.[124] Circulating levels of ceruloplasmin are positively correlated to levels of copper in the blood.[125,126] Increased levels of ceruloplasmin have been reported in AD brain compared with controls,[127,128] and both copper and ceruloplasmin levels have been shown to be elevated in the blood of patients with AD compared with controls.[129] This is consistent with our previous studies,[25] which showed that circulating ceruloplasmin levels were significantly and comparably increased in the AD, MCI, and low-function controls compared with the high function controls (see Figure 6.3). Copper ion has gained attention in AD because it may play a role in promoting production or toxicity of Aβ.[130–135]

Ceruloplasmin levels did not vary significantly in the placebo group during the ADCLT (see Figure 6.4). In contrast, circulating ceruloplasmin levels gradually decreased in the atorvastatin group, so that after 1 year of treatment there was a trend for reduced levels ($p = 0.07$) compared with levels identified at baseline (see Figure 6.4). An increase in circulating Aβ levels rather than a decrease with atorvastatin treatment was envisioned as a possibility in the ADCLT. This was based on the circulating ceruloplasmin levels identified in our cross-sectional studies of Brain Bank subjects (see Figure 6.3), coupled with our findings in cholesterol-fed rabbits. Slight gradual increases were observed (see Figure 6.5). Accumulation of Aβ is presumed to be a result of overproduction, but reduced clearance of the peptide is a likely contributing factor. Support for reduced clearance as a reason for central accumulation of Aβ comes from recent immunotherapy studies in transgenic mouse models of

AD, where introduction of $A\beta$ antibodies into the blood, which need not enter CNS proper, assist in the removal of $A\beta$ from the brain.[123,136] The mechanism by which atorvastatin treatment produced clinical benefit in AD patients remains elusive, but reduced influx of cholesterol into the brain, which results in reduced $A\beta$ production and enhanced efflux of existing $A\beta$, tends to be supported by data obtained in the ADCLT.

In 2002 Simons et al[99] reported the results of a randomized, double-blind placebo-controlled clinical trial of 44 AD patients treated with the BBB-permeable simvastatin (80 mg/day) or placebo for 26 weeks. Participants with an MMSE of 12–26 were recruited and 37 completed the study (20 simvastatin and 17 placebo). The groups were further stratified for analysis to those with mild (26–21) or more moderate (20–12) disease. When considering both the mild and moderate AD groups together, simvastatin treatment produced a significant decrease in circulating LDL-cholesterol, and, as noted above, a reduction in CSF $A\beta_{1-40}$ levels occurred among the mild but not the moderately affected participants. A significant benefit on MMSE performance, but not the ADAS-cog, was identified in the simvastatin-treated group compared with placebo at the end of the 26-week trial.

In the ADCLT we showed that at the first quarterly visit (13 weeks) there was deterioration in the MMSE (decreased score) and the ADAS-cog (increased score) similar to that seen in the placebo group, but by the second quarterly visit (26 weeks) there was improvement on the MMSE to the level of performance at entrance and improvement on the ADAS-cog to a level superior to the performance at trial entrance, whereas the placebo group deteriorated another point on each instrument.[20,89,113] This is consistent with an open-label study of 19 AD patients treated with simvastatin (20 mg/day) for 12 weeks, where there was an increase in ADAS-cog score (compared with baseline).[100] Our results are in part consistent with the results of Simons et al[99] for AD patients treated with simvastatin (80 mg/day) or placebo for 26 weeks. In both the ADCLT and Simons et al study the MMSE scores were almost identical prior to randomization and after 26 weeks of active treatment. In contrast, the placebo group deteriorated nearly 3 points on the MMSE in Simons et al's study, but only 1.5 points in the ADCLT. This resulted in a significant difference on the MMSE between the two groups at 26 weeks in the Simons et al study, but in the ADCLT the magnitude of the difference between the groups on the MMSE at 26 weeks was not sufficient to be significant. In contrast to the finding of Simons et al, keeping in mind the ADAS-cog is an error score, 26 weeks of atorvastatin treatment in the ADCLT produced an improvement on the ADAS-cog (–1.5 points) compared with baseline, whereas the placebo group deteriorated (2.5 points) compared with baseline. This produced a significant difference between the groups on the ADAS-cog ($p = 0.003$) at 26 weeks in the ADCLT. This was not the case in Simons et al study, where scores on the ADAS-cog deteriorated 4.1 points in the simvastatin-treated group and 3.4 points in the placebo group.[99] The difference in deterioration on the MMSE and ADAS-cog for the placebo groups between the ADCLT and

Simons et al study are somewhat curious in that participants had similar base-line performances and were of similar age at trial entrance. It will also be interesting to see if similar differences are observed for simvastatin and ator-vastatin in the ongoing multicenter AD treatment trials that are independently testing each medication, the CLASP and LEADe trials, respectively.

REFERENCES

1. Sparks DL, Hunsaker JC, Scheff SW, et al. Cortical senile plaques in coronary artery disease, aging and Alzheimer's disease. Neurobiol Aging 1990;11:601–607.

2. Sparks DL, Scheff SW, Hunsaker III JC, et al. Induction of Alzheimer-like β-amyloid immunoreactivity in the brains of rabbits with dietary choles-terol. Exp Neurol 1994;126:88–94.

3. Sparks DL, Connor DJ, Wasser DR, Lopez JE, Sabbagh MN. The Alzheimer's Disease Atorvastatin Treatment Trial: Scientific basis and position on the use of HMG-CoA reductase inhibitors (statins) that do or do not cross the blood–brain bar-rier. In: Advances in Drug Discovery and Drug Development for Cognitive Aging and Alzheimer's Disease. Berlin: Springer, 2000: 244–252.

4. Sparks DL, Martins R, Martin T. Cholesterol and cognition: rationale for the AD cholesterol-lowering treat-ment trial and sex-related differences in β-amyloid accumulation in the brains of spontaneously hyperchole-sterolemic Watanabe rabbits. Ann N Y Acad Sci 2002;977:356–366.

5. Bodovitz S, Klein WL. Cholesterol modulates alpha-secretase cleavage of amyloid precursor protein. J Biol Chem 1996;271(8):4436–4440.

6. Katzman R. A neurologist's view of Alzheimer's disease and dementia. Int Psychogeriatr 2004;16(3):259–273.

7. Miller LJ, Chacko R. The role of choles-terol and statins in Alzheimer's disease. Ann Pharmacother 2004;38(1):91–98.

8. Reiss AB, Siller KA, Rahman MM, et al. Cholesterol in neurologic dis-orders of the elderly: stroke and Alzheimer's disease. Neurobiol Aging 2004;25(8):977–989.

9. Teter B. ApoE-dependent plasticity in Alzheimer's disease. J Mol Neurosci 2004;23(3):167–179.

10. Burns M, Duff K. Cholesterol in Alzheimer's disease and tauopathy. Ann N Y Acad Sci 2002;977:367–375.

11. Wolozin B, Brown Jr, Theisler C, Silberman S. The cellular biochem-istry of cholesterol and statins: insights into pathophysiology and therapy of Alzheimer's disease. CNS Drug Rev 2004;10(2):126–146.

12. Poirier J. Apolipoprotein E and chol-esterol metabolism in the pathogene-sis treatment of Alzheimer's disease. Trends Mol Med 2003;9(3):94–101.

13. Kolsch H, Lutjohann D, von Bergmann K, Heun R. The role of 24S-hydroxycholesterol in Alzheimer's disease. J Nutr Health Aging 2003; 7(1):37–41.

14. Gibson Wood W, Eckert GP, Igbavboa U, Muller WE. Amyloid beta-protein interactions with membranes and cholesterol causes or casualties of Alzheimer's disease. Biochem Biophys Acta 2003;1610(2):281–290.

15. Michikawa M. Cholesterol paradox: is high total or low HDL cholesterol level a risk for Alzheimer's disease? J Neurosci Res 2003;72(2):141–146.

16. Caballero J, Nahata M. Do statins slow down Alzheimer's disease? A

review. J Clin Pharm Ther 2004; 29(3):209–213.

17. Michaelis ML. Drugs targeting Alzheimer's disease: some things old and some things new. J Pharmacol Exp Ther 2003;304(3):897–904.

18. Algotsson A, Winblad B. Patients with Alzheimer's disease may be particularly susceptible to adverse effects of statins. Dement Geriatr Cogn Disord 2004;17(3):109–116.

19. Jelic V, Winblad B. Treatment of mild cognitive impairment: rationale, present and future strategies. Acta Neurol Scand Suppl 2003;179:83–93.

20. Sparks DL, Connor D, Lopez J, et al. Benefit of atorvastatin in the treatment of Alzheimer's disease. Neurobiol Aging 2004;25(Suppl 1):S24.

21. Petersen RC, Stevens JC, Ganguli M, et al. Practice parameter: early detection of dementia: mild cognitive impairment (an evidence-based review). Report of the Quality Standard Subcommittee of the American Academy of Neurology. Neurology 2001;56:1133–1142.

22. Petersen RC, Smith GE, Waring SC, et al. Mild cognitive impairment. Clinical characterization and outcome. Arch Neurol 1999;56:303–308.

23. Schosinsky KH, Lehmann HP, Beeler MF. Measurment of ceruloplasmin from its oxidase activity in serum by the use of o-dianisidine dihydrochloride. Clin Chem 1974;20(12): 1556–1563.

24. Refolo LM, Malester B, LaFrancois J, et al. Hypercholesterolemia accelerates Alzheimer's amyloid pathology in a transgenic mouse model. Neurobiol Dis 2000;7(4):321–331.

25. Sparks DL, Petanceska S, Sabbagh M, et al. Cholesterol, copper and Aβ in controls, MCI, AD and the AD Cholesterol-Lowering Treatment trial (ADCLT). Curr Alz Res 2005; in press.

26. Folstein MF, Folstein SE, McHugh PR. "Mini-Mental State:" a practical method for grading the mental state of patients for the clinician. J Psychiatric Res 1975;12:189–198.

27. Rey A. L'examen Clinique en Psychologie. Paris: Presses Universitaires de France, 1964.

28. Borod JC, Goodglass H, Kaplan E. Normative data on the Boston Diagnostic Aphasia Examination, Parietal Lobe battery and the Boston Naming Test. J Clin Neuropsychol 1980;2:209–216.

29. Doty RL. The Smell Identification Test Administration Manual, 3rd edn. Haddon Heights, New Jersey: Sensonics, 1995.

30. Riemenschneider M, Lautenschlager N, Wagenpfeil S, et al. Cerebrospinal fluid tau and beta-amyloid 42 proteins identify Alzheimer disease in subjects with mild cognitive impairment. Arch Neurol 2002;59:1729–1734.

31. Maruyama M, Arai H, Sugita M, et al. Cerebrospinal fluid amyloid beta(1–42) levels in the mild cognitive impairment stage of Alzheimer's disease. Exp Neurol 2001;172: 433–436.

32. de Leon MJ, Segal S, Tarshish CY, et al. Longitudinal cerebrospinal fluid tau load increases in mild cognitive impairment. Neurosci Lett 2002;333: 183–186.

33. Parnetti L, Lanari A, Saggese E, Spaccatini C, Gallai V. Cerebrospinal fluid biochemical markers in early detection and differential diagnosis of dementia disorders in routine clinical practice. Neurol Sci 2003;24:199–200.

34. Fukumoto H, Tennis M, Locascio JJ, et al. Age but not diagnosis is the main predictor of plasma amyloid β protein levels. Arch Neurol 2003; 60(7):958–964.

35. Assini A, Cammarata S, Vitali A, et al. Plasma levels of amyloid beta-protein 42 are increased in women with mild cognitive impairment. Neurology 2004;63:828-831.

36. Prince M, Cullen M, Mann A. Risk factors for Alzheimer's disease and dementia: a case-control study based on the MRC elderly hypertension trial. Neurology 1994;44:97–104.

37. Breteler MM, Claus JJ, Grobbee DE, Hofman A. Cardiovascular disease and distribution of cognitive function in elderly people: the Rotterdam Study. BMJ 1994;308:1604–1608.

38. Wilson PWF, Myers RH, Larson MG, et al. Apolipoprotein E alleles, dyslipidemia and coronary heart disease. JAMA 1994;272:1666–1671.

39. Aronson MK, Ooi WL, Morgenstern H, et al. Women, myocardial infarction, and dementia in the very old. Neurology 1990;40:1102–1106.

40. Martins C, Gambert SR, Gupta KL, Schultz BM. Effect of age and dementia on the prevalence of cardiovascular disease. Age 1990;13:9–11.

41. Skoog I, Lernfelt B, Landahl S, et al. 15-year longitudinal study of blood pressure and dementia. Lancet 1996; 347:1141–1145.

42. Jarvik GP, Wijsman EM, Kukull WA, et al. Interactions of apolipoprotein E genotype, total cholesterol level, age, and sex in prediction of Alzheimer's disease: a case-control study. Neurology 1995;45:1092–1096.

43. Sparks DL. Coronary artery disease, hypertension, ApoE, and cholesterol: a link to Alzheimer's disease? Ann N Y Acad Sci 1997;826:128–146.

44. Grant WB. Dietary links to Alzheimer's disease. Alzheimer's Dis Rev 1997;2:42–55.

45. Desmond DW, Tatemichi TK, Paik M, Stern Y. Risk factors for cerebrovascular disease as correlates of cognitive function in a stroke-free cohort. Arch Neurol 1993;50:162–166.

46. Lehtonen A, Luutonen S. High-density lipoprotein cholesterol levels of very old people in the diagnosis of dementia. Age Ageing 1986;15: 267–270.

47. Giubilei F, D'Antona R, Antonini R, et al. Serum lipoprotein pattern variations in dementia and ischemic stroke. Acta Neurol Scand 1990;81: 84–86.

48. Czech C, Forstl H, Hentschel F, et al. Apolipoprotein E-4 gene dose in clinically diagnosed Alzheimer's disease: prevalence, plasma cholesterol levels and cerebrovascular change. Eur Arch Psychiatry Clin Neurosci 1994;243:291–292.

49. Mahieux F, Couderc R, Moulignier A, et al. Isoform 4 of apolipoprotein E and Alzheimer disease. Specificity and clinical study. Rev Neurol (Paris) 1995;151(4):231–239.

50. Kuo Y-M, Emmerling MR, Bisgaier CL, et al. Elevated low-density lipoprotein in Alzheimer's disease correlates with brain abeta 1-42 levels. Biochem Biophys Res Commun 1998;252(3):711–715.

51. Chandra V, Pandav R. Gene–environment interaction in Alzheimer's disease: a potential role for cholesterol. Neuroepidemiology 1998;17(5): 225–232.

52. Notkola IL, Sulkava R, Pekkanen J, et al. Serum total cholesterol, apolipoprotein E epsilon 4 allele, and Alzheimer's disease. Neuroepidemiology 1998;17: 14–20.

53. Olson RE. Discovery of the lipoproteins, their role in fat transport and their significance as risk factors. J Nutr 1998;128(2 Suppl):439S–443S.

54. Kalmijn S, Launer LJ, Ott A, et al. Dietary fat intake and the risk of incident dementia in the Rotterdam Study. Ann Neurol 1997;42:776–782.

55. Kuusisto J, Koivistom K, Mykkanen L, et al. Association between features of the insulin resistance syndrome and Alzheimer's disease independently of apolipoprotein E4 phenotype: cross sectional population based study. BMJ 1997;315:1045–1049.

56. Kivipelto M, Helkala E-L, Hallikainen M, et al. Elevated systolic

blood pressure and high cholesterol levels at midlife are risk factors for late-life dementia. Neurobiol Aging 2000;21(1S):S174.

57. Yasojima K, McGeer EG, McGeer PL. HMG Co-A reductase mRNA in AD and control brain. Neuroreport 2001; 12:2935–2938.

58. Sparks DL, Liu H, Gross DR, Scheff SW. Increased density of cortical apolipoprotein E immunoreactive neurons in rabbit brain after dietary administration of cholesterol. Neurosci Lett 1995;187:142-144.

59. Sparks DL. Intraneuronal β-amyloid immunoreactivity in the CNS. Neurobiol Aging 1996;17(2):291–299.

60. Sparks DL. Dietary cholesterol induces Alzheimer-like β-amyloid immunoreactivity in rabbit brain. Nutr Metab Cardiovasc Dis 1997; 7(3):255–266.

61. Streit WJ, Sparks DL. Activation of microglia in the brains of humans with heart disease and hypercholesterolemic rabbits. J Mol Med 1997;75:130–138.

62. Sparks DL. Neuropathologic links between Alzheimer's disease and vascular disease. In: Iqbal K, Swaab DF, Winblad B, Wisniewski HM, eds. Alzheimer's Disease and Related Disorders. Chichester, UK: John Wiley & Sons, 1999: 153–163.

63. Sparks DL, Kou Y-M, Roher A, Martin TA, Lukas RJ. Alterations of Alzheimer's disease in the cholesterol-fed rabbit, including vascular inflammation. Preliminary observations. NY Acad Sci 2000;903: 335–344.

64. Fishman CE, White SL, DeLong CA, et al. High fat diet potentiates β-amyloid deposition in the APP V717F transgenic mouse model of Alzheimer's disease. Soc Neurosci 1999;25:1859.

65. Bales KR, Fishman C, DeLong C, et al. Diet-induced hyperlipidemia accelerates amyloid deposition in the APPv717f transgenic mouse model of Alzheimer's disease. Neurobiol Aging 2000;21(1S):S139.

66. Shie F-G, Jin L-W, Cook DG, Leverenz JB, LeBoeul RC. Diet-induced hypercholesterolemia enhances brain Aβ accumulation in transgenic mice. NeuroReport 2002; 13:455–459.

67. Levin-Allerhand JA, Lominska CE, Smith JD. Increased amyloid levels in APPSWE transgenic mice treated chronically with a physiological high-fat high-cholesterol diet. J Nutr Health Aging 2002;6:315–319.

68. Racchi M, Baetta R, Salvietti N, et al. Secretory processing of amyloid precursor protein is inhibited by increase in cellular cholesterol content. Biochem J 1997;322:893–898.

69. Simons M, Keller P, De Strooper B, et al. Cholesterol depletion inhibits the generation of beta-amyloid in hippocampal neurons. Proc Natl Acad Sci USA 1998;95(11):6460–6464.

70. Frears ER, Stephens DJ, Walters CE, Davies H, Austen BM. The role of cholesterol in the biosynthesis of β-amyloid. NeuroReport 1999;10: 1699–1705.

71. Galbete JL, Martin TR, Peressini E, et al. Cholesterol decreases secretion of the secreted form of amyloid precursor protein by interfering with glycosylation in the protein secretory pathway. Biochem J 2000;348(Pt 2):307–313.

72. Austen BM, Frears ER, Davies H. Cholesterol upregulates production of Abeta 1–40 and 1–42 in transfected cells. Neurobiol Aging 2000; 21(1S):S254.

73. Beyreuther K. Physiological function of APP processing. Neurobiol Aging 2000;21(1S):S69.

74. Urmoneit B, Turner J, Dyrks T. Cationic lipids (lipofectamine) and disturbance of cellular cholesterol and sphingomyelin distribution modulates gamma-secretase activity with-

in amyloid precursor protein in vitro. Prostaglandins Other Lipid Mediat 1998;55(5–6):331–343.

75. Kirsch C, Eckert GP, Koudinov AR, Muller WE. Brain cholesterol, statins and Alzheimer's disease. Pharmacopsychiatry 2003;36)Suppl 2):s113–s119.

76. Bergmann C, Runz H, Jakala P, Hartmann T. Diversification of gamma-secretase versus beta-secretase inhibition by cholesterol depletion. Neurobiol Aging 2000; 21(1S):S278.

77. Fassbender K, Simons M, Bergmann C, et al. Simvastatin strongly reduces levels of Alzheimer's disease beta-amyloid peptides Abeta 42 and Abeta 40 in vitro and in vivo. Prco Natl Acad Sci USA 2001;98(10):5856–5861.

78. Michikawa M, Yanagisawa K. Apolipoprotein E4 induces neuronal cell death under conditions of suppressed de novo cholesterol synthesis. J Neurosci Res 1998;54(1):58–67.

79. Sparks DL, Connor DJ, Browne PJ, Lopez JE, Sabbagh MN. HMG-CoA reductase inhibitors (statins) in the treatment of Alzheimer's disease and why it would be ill-advised to use one that crosses the blood–brain barrier. J Nutr Health Aging 2002; 6(5):324–331.

80. Refolo LM, Pappolla MA, LaFrancois J, et al. A cholesterol-lowering drug reduces beta-amyloid pathology in a transgenic mouse model of Alzheimer's disease. Neurobiol Dis 2001;5:890–899.

81. Petanceska SS, DeRosa S, Olm V, et al. Statin therapy for Alzheimer's disease. Will it work? J Mol Neurosci 2002;19:155–161.

82. Park IH, Hwang EM, Hong HS, et al. Lovastatin enhances Abeta production and senile plaque deposits in female Tf2576 mice. Neurobiol Aging 2003;24(5):637–643.

83. Chauhan N, Siegel G, Feinstein D. Effects of lovastatin and pravastatin on amyloid processing and inflammatory response in TgCRND8 brain. Neurochem Res 2004;29(10):1897–1911.

84. Petanceska S, Pappolla M, Refolo M. Modulation of Alzheimer's amyloidosis by statins: mechanisms of action. Crit Rev Med Chem 2003;3:1–7.

85. Puglielli L, Konopaka G, Pack-Chung E, et al. Acyl-coenzyme A: cholesterol acyltransferase modulates the generation of the amyloid beta-peptide. Nat Cell Biol 2001;3(10): 905–912.

86. Puglielli L, Tanzi RE, Kovacs DM. Alzheimer's disease: the cholesterol connection. Nature Neurosci 2003; 6(4):345–351.

87. Puglielli L, Ellis BC, Ingano LA, Kovacs DM. Role of acyl-coenzyme A: cholesterol acyltransferase activity in the processing of the amyloid precursor protein. J Mol Neurosci 2004;24:93–96.

88. Sun YX, Crisby M, Lindgren S, Janciauskiene S. Pravastatin inhibits pro-inflammatory effects of Alzheimer's peptide Abeta (1-42) in glioma cell culture in vitro. Pharmacol Res 2003;47(2):119–126.

89. Sparks DL, Sabbagh MN, Connor DJ, et al. Atorvastatin therapy lowers circulating cholesterol but not free radical activity in advance of identifiable clinical benefit in the treatment of mild-to-moderate AD. Curr AD Res 2005;2:343–353.

90. Hill J, Steiner I, Matthews K, et al. Statins lower the risk of developing Alzheimer's disease by limiting lipid raft endocytosis and decreasing the neuronal spread of Herpes simplex virus type 1. Med Hypotheses 2005; 64(1):53–58.

91. Vega GL, Weiner MF, Lipton AM, et al. Reduction in levels of 24S-hydroxycholesterol by statin treatment in patients with Alzheimer disease. Arch Neurol 2003;60:510–515.

92. Petanceska SS, DeRosa S, Sharma A, et al. Changes in apolipoprotein E

expression in response to dietary and pharmacological modulation of cholesterol. J Mol Neurosci 2003;20(3): 395–406.

93. Pedrini S, Carter TL, Prendergast G, et al. Modulation of statin-activiated shedding of alzheimer APP ectodomain by ROCK. PLoS Med 2005;2:1–12.

94. Friedhoff LT, Cullen EI, Geoghagen NS, Buxbaum JD. Treatment with controlled-release lovastatin decreases serum concentrations of human beta-amyloid (A beta) peptide. Int J Neuropsychopharmacol 2001;4: 127–130.

95. Buxbaum JD, Cullen EI, Friedhoff LT. Pharmacological concentrations of the HMG-CoA reductase inhibitor lovastatin decrease the formation of the Alzheimer beta-amyloid peptide in vitro and in patients. Front Biosci 2002;7:a50–a59.

96. Tokuda T, Takaoka A, Matsuno S, et al. Plasma levels of amyloid beta did not differ between subjects taking statins and those not taking statins. Ann Neurol 2001;49:546–547.

97. Hoglund K, Wikiund O, Vanderstichele H, et al. Plasma levels of beta-amyloid(1–40), beta-amyloid(1–42), and total beta-amyloid remain unaffected in adult patients with hypercholesterolemia after treatment with statins. Arch Neurol 2004; 61:333–337.

98. Ishii K, Tokuda T, Matsushima T, et al. Pravastatin at 10 mg/day does not decrease plasma levels of either amyloid-beta (Abeta) 40 or Abeta 42 in humans. Neurosci Lett 2003;350(3): 161–164.

99. Simons M, Schwarzler F, Lutjohann D, et al. Treatment with simvastatin in normocholesterolemic patients with Alzheimer's disease: a 26-week, randomized, placebo controlled, double-blind trial. Ann Neurol 2002;52: 346–350.

100. Sjogren M, Gustafsson K, Syversen S, et al. Treatment with simvastatin in

patients with Alzheimer's disease lowers both alpha- and beta-cleaved amyloid precursor protein. Dement Geriatr Cogn Disord 2003;16(1): 25–30.

101. Wolozin B, Kellman W, Ruosseau P, Celesia G, Siegel G. Decreased prevalence of Alzheimer disease associated with 3-hydroxy-3-methylglutaryl coenzyme A reductase inhibitors. Arch Neurol 2000;57(10):1439– 1443.

102. Jick H, Zornberg G, Jick S, Seshadri S, Drachman D. Statins and the risk of dementia. Lancet 2000;56(9242): 1627–1631.

103. Rodriguez E, Dodge H, Birzescu M, Stoehr G, Ganguli M. Use of lipid-lowering drugs in older adults with and without dementia: a community-based epidemiological study. J Am Geriatr Soc 2002;50(11):1852–1856.

104. Yaffe K, Barrett-Connor E, Lin F, Grady D. Serum lipoprotein levels, statin use, and cognitive function in older women. Arch Neurol 2002;59:378–384.

105. Rockwood K, Kirkland S, Hogan DB, et al. Use of lipid-lowering agents, indication bias, and the risk of dementia in community-dwelling elderly people. Arch Neurol 2002; 59:223–227.

106. Zamrini E, McGwin G, Roseman JM. Association between statin use and Alzheimer's disease. Neuroepidemiology 2004;23(1–2):94–98.

107. Starr J, McGurn B, Whiteman M, et al. Life long changes in cognitive ability are associated with prescription medications in old age. Int J Geriatr Psychiatry 2004;19(4):327– 332.

108. Li G, Higdon R, Kukull W, et al. Statin therapy and risk of dementia in the elderly: a community based prospective cohort study. Neurology 2004;63(9):1624–1628.

109. Zandi PP, Sparks DL, Khachaturian AS, et al. Do statins reduce risk of incident dementia and Alzheimer

disease? The Cache County Study. Arch Gen Psychiatry 2005;62(2): 217–224.

110. Lutjohann D, von Bergmann K. 24S-hydroxycholesterol: a marker of brain cholesterol metabolism. Pharmacopsychiatry 2003;36 (Suppl 2):s102–s106.

111. Baskin F, Rosenberg RN, Fang X, et al. Correlation of statin-increased platelet APP ratios and reduced lipids in AD patients. Neurology 2003; 60(12):2006–2007.

112. Doraiswamy PM, Steffens DC, McQuoid DR. Statin use and hippocampal volumes in elderly subjects at risk for Alzheimer's disease: a pilot observational study. Am J Alzheimers Dis Other Demen 2004;19(5): 275–278.

113. Sparks DL, Sabbagh MN, Connor DJ, et al. Atorvastatin for the treatment of mild-to-moderate Alzheimer's disease: preliminary results. Arch Neurol 2005;62(5):753–757.

114. Rosen WG, Mohs RC, Davis KL. A new rating scale for Alzheimer's disease. Am J Psychiatry 1984;141(11): 1356–1364.

115. Kaufer DI, Cummings JL, Christine D, et al. Assessing the impact of neuropsychiatric symptoms in Alzheimer's disease: The Neuropsychiatric Inventory Caregiver Distress Scale. J Am Geriatr Soc 1998;46:210–215.

116. Schneider LS, Olin JT, Doody RS, et al. Validity and reliability of the Alzheimer's Disease Cooperative Study – Clinical Global Impression of Change. The Alzheimer's Disease Cooperative Study. Alzheimer Dis Assoc Disord 1997;11(Suppl 2):S22–S32.

117. Galasko D, Corey-Bloom J, Thal LJ. Monitoring progression in Alzheimer's disease. J Am Geriatr Soc 1991;39(9):932–941.

118. Galasko D, Bennett D, Sano M, et al. An inventory to assess activities of daily living for clinical trials in Alzheimer's disease. The Alzheimer's Disease Cooperative Study. Alzheimer Dis Assoc Disord 1997;11(Suppl 2):S33–S39.

119. Yesavage JA. Geriatric Depression Scale. Psychopharmacol Bull 1988; 24(4):709–711.

120. Sparks DL, Lochhead J, Horstman D, Wagoner T, Martin T. Water quality has a pronounced effect on cholesterol-induced accumulation of Alzheimer amyloid β (Aβ) in rabbit brain. J Alzheimers Dis 2002;4:523–529.

121. Sparks DL, Schreurs BG. Trace amounts of copper in water induce β-amyloid plaques and learning deficits in a rabbit model of Alzheimer's disease. Proc Natl Acad Sci USA 2003;100(19):1065–1069.

122. DeMattos RB, Bales KR, Parsadanian M, et al. Plaque-associated disruption of CSF and plasma amyloid-beta (Abeta) equilibrium in a mouse model of Alzheimer's disease. J Neurochem 2002;81(2):229–236.

123. DeMattos RB, Bales KR, Cummins DJ, Paul SM, Holtzman DM. Brain to plasma amyloid-beta efflux: a measure of brain amyloid burden in a mouse model of Alzheimer's disease. Science 2002;295:2264–2267.

124. Waggoner DJ, Bartnikas TB, Gitlin JD. The role of copper in neurodegenerative disease. Neurobiol Dis 1999;6:221–230.

125. Iskra M, Majewski W. Copper and zinc concentration and the activities of ceruloplasmin and superoxide dismutatse in atherosclerosis obliterans. Biol Trace Elem Res 2000;73:55–65.

126. Piorunska-Stolzman M, Iskra M, Majewski W. The activity of cholesterol esterase and ceruloplasmin are inversely related in the serum of men with atherosclerosis obliterans. Med Sci Monit 2001;7:940–945.

127. Wang H, Yu M, Ochani M, et al. Nicotinic acetylcholine receptor alpha7 subunit is an essential regulator of inflammation. Nature 2003; 421(6921):384–388.

128. Parakh N, Gupta HL, Jain A. Evaluation of enzymes in serum and cerebrospinal fluid in cases of stroke. Neurol India 2002;50:518–519.

129. Squitti R, Lupoi D, Pasqualetti P, et al. Elevation of serum copper levels in Alzheimer's disease. Neurology 2002;59(8):1153–1161.

130. Huang X, Cuajungco MP, Atwood CS, et al. Alzheimer's disease, beta-amyloid protein and zinc. J Nutr 2000;130(5S Suppl):1488S–1492S.

131. Cuajungco MP, Goldstein LE, Nunomura A, et al. Evidence that the beta-amyloid plaques of Alzheimer's disease represent the redox-silencing and entombment of Abeta by zinc. J Biol Chem 2000;275(26): 19439–19442.

132. Moir RD, Atwood CS, Romano DM, et al. Differential effects of apolipoprotein E isoforms on metal-induced aggregation of A beta using physiological concentrations. Biochemistry 1999; 38(14):4595–4603.

133. Chen M, Durr J, Fernandez HL. Possible role of calpain in normal processing of beta-amyloid precursor protein in human platelets. Biochem Biophys Res Commun 2000;273(1): 170–175.

134. White AR, Reyes R, Mercer JF, et al. Copper levels are increased in the cerebral cortex and liver of APP and APLP2 knockout mice. Brain Res 1999;842(2):439–444.

135. Atwood CS, Scarpa RC, Huang X, et al. Characterization of copper interactions with Alzheimer amyloid beta peptides: Identification of an atto-molar-affinity copper binding site on amyloid beta1–42. J Neurochem 2000;75(3):1219–1233.

136. DeMattos RB, Bales KR, Cummins DJ, et al. Peripheral anti-A beta antibody alters CNS and plasma A beta clearance and decreases brain A beta burden in a mouse model of Alzheimer's disease. Proc Natl Acad Sci USA 2001;98(15):8850–8855.

7
Insulin resistance in Alzheimer's disease – a novel therapeutic target

Suzanne Craft, Mark A Reger, and Laura D Baker

INTRODUCTION

The search for risk factors that increase the risk of Alzheimer's disease (AD) has converged on a cluster of disorders characterized by vascular, lipid, and metabolic abnormalities, such as cardiovascular disease, hypertension, and type 2 diabetes mellitus (T2DM). A common pathophysiology uniting these diseases is derangement of insulin metabolism, characterized by the inability of insulin to efficiently promote glucose uptake into muscle (insulin resistance), with concomitant peripheral insulin elevations (hyperinsulinemia). Although much attention has been paid to the metabolic consequences of insulin resistance, peripheral hyperinsulinemia has additional deleterious effects on systems that do not habituate to increased insulin. For example, as will be discussed, peripheral hyperinsulinemia has effects on inflammation and brain insulin levels that are of special relevance to the pathogenesis of AD. There are probably several pathways leading to the final common expression of AD pathology.[1] Insulin resistance and peripheral hyperinsulinemia comprise one potential pathway, and as such do not apply to all AD patients. It is, however, a pathway with relevance to a rapidly growing segment of our population. Peripheral hyperinsulinemia and insulin resistance are mutually reinforcing (each can cause or exacerbate the other) and may result from a number of causes, including genetic vulnerability and/or environmental factors such as diet and inactivity. They are also increasingly common conditions, in part due to the complexity of insulin signaling pathways, and in part due to pervasive changes in diet and physical activity occurring at an unprecedented rate in Western societies. In this chapter, we discuss mechanisms through which insulin resistance and peripheral hyperinsulinemia may induce AD pathogenesis, and the manner in which greater understanding of these mechanisms may lead to the development of novel therapeutic strategies.

INSULIN ACTION IN THE BRAIN

Until recently, insulin's actions in the brain were unclear. Although peripheral insulin readily crosses the blood–brain barrier (BBB) by a saturable, receptor-mediated process,[2–4] controversy persists as to whether insulin is synthesized within the central nervous system (CNS). Nonetheless, insulin is clearly active in the CNS, and the presence of insulin in the brain has been irrevocably confirmed using experimental methods of biochemical assay and mRNA detection.[5–9] Insulin receptors are located in the synapses of astrocytes and neurons,[10] and are found in high concentrations in the choroid plexus, olfactory bulb, piriform cortex, amygdala, hippocampus, hypothalamic nucleus, cerebellum, and cerebral cortex.[11–16]

In-vitro and in-vivo studies provide strong evidence for a link between insulin action and memory. Numerous insulin receptors are found in brain regions that play a critical role in the formation of new memories including the hippocampus and medial temporal cortex. Insulin improves passive-avoidance learning following intracerebroventricular administration in rats,[15] and verbal recall following intravenous infusion (maintaining euglycemia) in humans.[17–20] Interestingly, memory processes may exert reciprocal effects on insulin actions as well. Zhao and colleagues reported learning-induced increases in insulin receptor expression and tyrosine phosphorylation, implicating effects not only on insulin receptor distribution but also on insulin signaling in the hippocampus of rats who received training on a water maze task.[21]

Although normal actions of insulin may be beneficial for memory function, chronic peripheral hyperinsulinemia and insulin resistance may have a negative influence. Persistently elevated peripheral insulin levels have deleterious effects on BBB insulin receptors and, consequently, transport of insulin into the CNS.[22,23] In animal and human studies, peripheral insulin abnormalities, commonly associated with T2DM, are linked to impaired learning in animal and in human studies.[24] Impairments in verbal memory, in particular, have been noted for adults with chronic hyperinsulinemia without hyperglycemia,[25] and for adults with impaired glucose tolerance with concomitant increased hippocampal atrophy.[26] The results of these studies suggest that acute elevations in insulin play a salutary role in normal memory function, whereas persistent elevations are probably detrimental. Together, these divergent effects of acute and chronic hyperinsulinemia on memory provide further evidence for a clear link between insulin action and memory function.

Potential mechanisms underlying this link between insulin and memory include insulin's ability to modulate cerebral energy metabolism, critical neurophysiologic processes, and CNS neurotransmitter levels integral for cognitive function. Insulin does not appear to have a direct effect on transport of glucose into the brain, but rather on metabolism of cerebral glucose in selective brain circuits. In fact, low-dose peripheral insulin administration is associated with increased glucose metabolism, as measured by positron emission tomography (PET) using [^{18}F]fluorodeoxyglucose (FDG), particularly in cortical regions. This finding implicates a contributory role of insulin in the regulation of brain glucose uptake.[27] Regional differences in glucose metabolism may relate to the distribution pattern of insulin-sensitive glucose transporter isoforms (GLUTs),[28,29] such as GLUT 4 and GLUT 8, which each have distinct kinetic properties to permit precise region-specific metabolic regulation. In rats, GLUT 4 is expressed in motor areas, hippocampus, pituitary, and hypothalamus.[30–33] GLUT 8 expression has been documented in hippocampus, hypothalamus, and cerebral cortex.[28] Co-localized distributions of insulin-containing neurons, insulin receptors, and GLUTs 4 and 8[29,30] in these areas suggest a role for insulin in region-specific regulation of glucose metabolism, particularly in medial temporal lobe structures that support learning and memory.

In addition to this glucoregulatory role, insulin affects physiologic processes at the cellular and molecular levels within the same brain regions that are essential for new memory formation.[34] For example, insulin modulates components of the long-term potentiation cascade, affecting processes associated with neurotransmitter release at presynaptic terminals, as well as activities at postsynaptic sites involving NMDA (N-methyl-D-aspartate) and GABA (γ-aminobutyrate) receptors.[34,35] At the molecular level, insulin activates specific signaling pathways that are associated with memory formation. Thus, insulin's role in CNS function involves a host of mechanisms, extending from region-specific glucose regulation to actions that impact neurochemical and neurophysiologic cellular processes in brain areas known to support memory function.

INSULIN ABNORMALITIES AND ALZHEIMER'S DISEASE RISK

Population-based epidemiologic studies link impaired insulin function to increased risk of developing AD in older adults. Although not undisputed, this link is supported by studies that clinically evaluated diabetes, hyperinsulinemia, and insulin resistance using standard diagnostic procedures such as oral glucose tolerance testing, as well as neuroimaging techniques to more effectively differentiate AD from vascular dementia. When insulin abnormalities and AD pathology are carefully characterized in this way, risk of either AD or vascular dementia is clearly increased for older adults with diabetes and insulin resistance. This association is supported by two large prospective, population-based cohort studies, the Rotterdam Study[36] and the Honolulu–Asia Aging Study.[37] Interestingly, Leibson and colleagues[38] found that even though hyperinsulinemia increases risk for dementia overall, it increases risk for AD to an even greater extent. Mayeaux and colleagues provide additional confirmation for this link between diabetes, hyperinsulinemia, and AD risk. In their prospective community-based study, memory scores declined faster over time and the risk of AD doubled among hyperinsulinemic adults, a group that constituted 39% of the total sample of 683 older adults.[39] Finally, the results of other cross-sectional and prospective studies support an association between increased fasting plasma insulin levels and increased AD prevalence and incidence, as well as evidence to suggest faster memory decline regardless of diabetic status. Overall, the implications of these data are that insulin resistance, independent of diabetes, may increase risk of developing AD.[40]

INSULIN ABNORMALITIES AND ALZHEIMER'S DISEASE PATHOLOGY

The manner in which insulin abnormalities may contribute to the symptoms and pathogenesis of AD have been examined in a variety of experimental models. Hoyer and colleagues were the first group to suggest that desensitization of the neuronal insulin receptor plays a role in AD.[41] In support of this theory, they have demonstrated a reduction in insulin receptors and tyrosine kinase activity markers in AD brain.[42]

Animal and in-vitro studies have documented relationships between insulin and mechanisms with clear pathogenic implications for AD. In vitro, insulin modulates levels of the amyloid beta (Aβ) peptide, the aggregation of which is a fundamental neuropathologic hallmark of AD. For example, insulin promotes release of intracellular Aβ in neuronal cultures, affecting both its short ($A\beta_{40}$) and long ($A\beta_{42}$) forms and accelerating their trafficking from the Golgi and trans-Golgi network to the plasma membrane.[43] Thus, low brain insulin may reduce the release of Aβ from intracellular to extracellular compartments. A growing understanding of the importance of impaired Aβ clearance, as opposed to increased Aβ production in late-onset AD, has created intense focus on mechanisms regulating Aβ degradation. Insulin may modulate Aβ degradation by regulating expression of insulin-degrading enzyme (IDE), a metalloprotease that catabolizes insulin.[44] IDE is highly expressed in brain as well as in liver, kidney, and muscle,[45] and may play a critical role in Aβ clearance in brain.[40,46,47] IDE has also been implicated in the regulation of intracellular degradation of Aβ, as compared with the neutral endopeptidase neprilysin.[48] Several studies have provided evidence that *IDE* gene polymorphisms may be related to hyperinsulinemia, AD, and Aβ levels. Association of AD with a locus on chromosome 10 in the region of the *IDE* gene has been identified in several, but not all, studies.[49–54] Furthermore, decreased IDE activity, levels, and mRNA have been observed in AD brain tissue, and IDE knockout mice have reduced degradation of Aβ and insulin in brain.[55–57] Thus, low CNS insulin may reduce IDE levels in brain and thereby impair Aβ clearance. Conversely, excessively high insulin levels may act as a competitive substrate for IDE and inhibit its degradation of Aβ.

Low brain insulin levels in AD may be due in part to chronic peripheral hyperinsulinemia, which may also interfere with peripheral Aβ clearance. Chronic peripheral hyperinsulinemia has been associated with a pattern in which brain insulin levels are initially higher, then decrease as transport of insulin into the brain is down-regulated.[58] Consistent with this pattern, it has been shown that genetically obese Zucker rats have reduced insulin binding to brain capillaries[59] and reduced hypothalamic insulin levels[60] in comparison with lean controls. Additionally, in an elegant study in which insulin resistance was induced in dogs through diet, brain uptake of labeled insulin was reduced and peripheral insulin clearance was inhibited.[61] We have documented that patients with AD have lower cerebrospinal fluid (CSF) insulin levels, higher plasma insulin levels, and reduced CSF-to-plasma insulin ratios compared with healthy controls.[62] High plasma insulin levels may interfere with degradation of Aβ transported out of the brain, thereby obstructing a peripheral Aβ-clearing 'sink'. Concomitantly, low brain insulin levels reduce release of Aβ from intracellular compartments into extracellular compartments, where clearance is believed to occur. Thus, for some patients with AD, high peripheral insulin levels and low brain insulin levels would result in reduced clearance of Aβ both in brain and in the periphery.

Support for the validity of this model is provided by a recent study that induced insulin resistance in the T2576 mouse model of AD with a high fat diet. Diet manipulation resulted in a metabolic profile of high peripheral insulin, and low brain insulin and IDE levels, compared with Tg2576 mice fed a normal diet.[63] Diet-induced insulin resistance caused twofold increases in $A\beta_{40}$ and $A\beta_{42}$ in brain, and earlier, larger Aβ deposits compared with non-insulin-resistant mice. Furthermore, insulin-resistant mice had impaired learning on a water maze test. These results are consistent with recent evidence that insulin regulates IDE and Aβ through a phosphatidylinositol-3-kinase-dependent signaling mechanism.[44] Treatment of primary hippocampal neurons with insulin produced a 25% increase in IDE expression. Together, these results suggest that insulin resistance can precipitate the neuropathologic and behavioral features of AD, and that raising brain insulin levels may reduce neuropathologic changes related to AD.

One mechanism that may affect both insulin and IDE function is excessive or chronic glucocorticoid elevation. The antagonistic effects of the glucocorticoid cortisol on insulin-mediated glucose transport have been well-documented. Hypercortisolemia appears to interfere with intracellular signaling mechanisms and to reduce the population of insulin receptors capable of undergoing tyrosine phosphorylation, in addition to reducing expression of insulin receptor substrate 1 (IRS1).[64] Glucocorticoids have been shown to reduce expression and activity of IDE. Glucocorticoid receptor fragments bind to IDE and inhibit its insulin-degrading capacity in vitro.[65] Glucocorticoid treatment has also been associated with a reduction in the insulin-degrading capacity of hepatocytes in culture.[66] Furthermore, glucocorticoids can inhibit the ability of insulin to bind to IDE, a process thought to be essential for normal signaling to occur.[67] Peripheral administration of the glucocorticoid dexamethasone reduced insulin transport into CNS in an in-vivo dog model.[68] In a recent study, we showed that inducing hypercortisolemia for 1 year in aged macaques reduced IDE levels and increased $A\beta_{42}$ levels in brain[69] (Figure 7.1). Taken together, these results suggest that hypercortisolemia may interfere with insulin's ability to regulate IDE levels in brain, either by decreasing CNS insulin availability or impeding its signaling efficacy. This possibility has important implications for models of AD pathogenesis, given that increased peripheral glucocorticoid levels have been consistently documented for patients with AD,[70–74] in older adults with the apoE-ε4 allele,[75] and in an animal model of AD.[76] In addition, we have shown that IDE protein levels are reduced in the brains of AD patients with the ε4 allele, who are most likely to have hypercortisolemia[55] (Figure 7.2).

Another potential mechanism involving insulin that has clear pathogenic implications for AD involves the hormone's ability to influence phosphorylation of tau, the constituent protein in the neurofibrillary lesions associated with AD, and to promote tau binding to microtubules through its actions on a downstream target in the insulin signaling pathway, glycogen synthase kinase

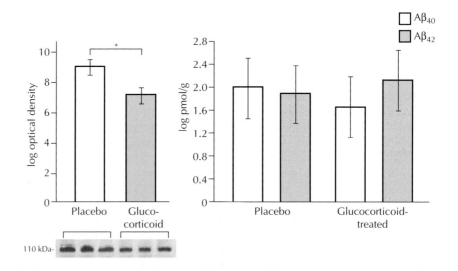

Figure 7.1

Western blots for insulin-degrading enzyme (IDE) (**A**) and amyloid beta (Aβ) (**B**) protein levels in the inferior frontal cortex. Image displays representative bands from three different subjects in both the placebo and glucocorticoid-treated groups. Graphs present the mean IDE (**A**) and $A\beta_{40}$ and $A\beta_{42}$ levels (**B**) ± SEM in primates exposed to 12 months of high-dose glucocorticoid (5.78 mg/kg/day hydrocortisone acetate) or placebo. Reduced IDE levels in the inferior frontal cortex are associated with glucocorticoid treatment (*$p < 0.05$). $A\beta_{42}$ was increased and $A\beta_{40}$ levels decreased in the glucocorticoid-treated animals ($p < 0.05$).

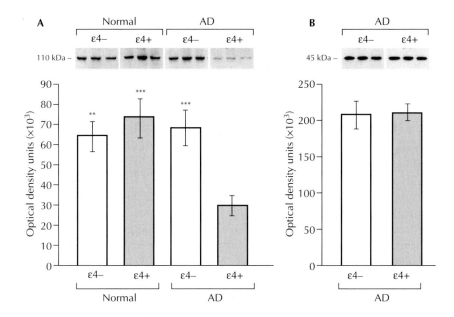

Figure 7.2

Quantitative Western blot analysis of hippocampal insulin-degrading enzyme (IDE)
(**A**) and neuron-specific enolase (NSE) (**B**) protein expression. Representative
immunoblots contain 100 μg (IDE) or 4 μg (NSE) of protein per lane from three
normal and/or three Alzheimer's disease (AD) subjects without (ε4–) and with
(ε4+) the APOE-ε4 allele. Graphs represent quantitative differences in expression of
IDE protein in normal and AD subjects (**A**) and of NSE protein in AD subjects (**B**)
with and without the ε4 allele. Each bar represents the mean ± SEM. IDE protein is
reduced in AD patients with an APOE-ε4 allele compared to patients without the
ε4 allele (***, $p = 0.0008$), to normal adults with the _4 allele (***, $p = 0.0004$),
and to normal adults without the ε4 allele (**, $p = 0.0011$). No differences in NSE
levels were observed for the AD groups ($p = 0.89$).

(GSK)-3.[77] GSK-3 phosphorylates tau in vitro[78,79] and in non-neuronal cells
transfected with tau.[80,81] The activity of GSK-3 and its isoforms GSK 3α and β,
can be down-regulated in response to insulin or insulin-like growth factor-1
(IGF-1) through the activation of the phosphatidylinositol 3-kinase pathway.
Schubert and colleagues[82] recently found that neuron-specific insulin receptor
knockout (NIRKO) mice exhibit a complete loss of insulin-mediated activation of this pathway, significantly reduced Akt and GSK 3β phosphorylation
and, consequently, increased phosphorylation of tau in excess of threefold.
Recent work also implicates insulin receptor substrate 2 (IRS2) proteins in the
pathogenic AD process. Normally, IRS2 protects the aging brain from phosphorylated tau accumulation. However, IRS2 knockout mice showed a marked
increase in tau phosphorylation and in tangle production.[83] Other pathogenic
mechanisms involving insulin, listed earlier, include its influence on

neurotransmitter levels, cerebral glucose metabolism, and cell membrane physiology, particularly in brain regions supporting learning and memory. Finally, interactions involving insulin abnormalities and oxidative stress, inflammation, and impaired neurogenesis[84] are likely culprits contributing to pathogenic processes of AD.

A MODEL OF PERIPHERAL HYPERINSULINEMIA, INSULIN RESISTANCE, AND ALZHEIMER'S DISEASE PATHOGENESIS

In the preceding sections, we have reviewed evidence supporting the notion that high plasma insulin levels and peripheral insulin resistance can affect CNS insulin levels, cognition, and $A\beta_{42}$ in the CNS. From such evidence a model can be constructed to describe how this metabolic profile contributes to the pathogenesis of AD.

The first component of our model concerns the effects of chronic peripheral hyperinsulinemia and insulin resistance on brain insulin levels. Peripheral hyperinsulinemia and insulin resistance down-regulate brain insulin uptake at the BBB, resulting in long-term reduction of brain insulin levels.[58–61] This phenomenon has been modeled in vivo in dogs with diet and glucocorticoid-induced insulin resistance[61,68] and was also observed in diet-induced insulin-resistant Tg 2576 mice (G Pasinetti, pers comm). Furthermore, we presented evidence above that patients with AD have lower CSF insulin levels, higher plasma insulin levels, and reduced CSF-to-plasma insulin ratios compared with healthy controls.[62] Given that insulin promotes the release of intracellular $A\beta$,[85] and regulates expression of IDE levels,[44] abnormally low brain insulin levels may result in increased intraneuronal accumulation of $A\beta$ and reduced levels of a protease that plays a major role in its clearance. Lowered brain insulin also has effects that may not be directly related to $A\beta$ regulation, such as decreased neurotransmitters and energy availability, increased oxidative stress and tau hyperphosphorylation, and reduced capacity for injury repair, synaptic remodeling, and neurogenesis.

A second component of our model relates to the effects of peripheral hyperinsulinemia in AD, which may inhibit the clearance of $A\beta_{42}$ from the brain into the periphery.[86] The obstruction of this peripheral 'sink' can presumably occur either by blocking $A\beta$ transport from brain, or by interfering with $A\beta$ clearance in peripheral sites, and as a result may promote excessive brain $A\beta_{42}$ accumulation. There may be several sites of peripheral $A\beta$ clearance. For example, the liver has been proposed as one of the primary clearance sites.[87] Low levels of insulin promote $A\beta$ clearance in a liver cell line under normal metabolic conditions.[88] Hepatic insulin resistance such as has been associated with prolonged hyperinsulinemia and glucocorticoid elevations may thus interfere with this process. Conversely, chronic or extreme insulin elevations may inhibit peripheral $A\beta$ clearance, in part because high insulin levels compete for the attention of IDE, the protease believed to play a major role in Aβ degradation, that is highly expressed in peripheral sites such as liver, kidney, and muscle. Insulin resistance also inhibits IDE activity, further contributing to decreased Aβ clearance. Thus, the combined effects of insulin resistance and hyperinsulinemia in liver and other peripheral sites may reduce Aβ uptake and degradation, leading to the high levels of plasma $Aβ_{42}$ documented in some AD patients.[89] Recent findings suggest that plasma Aβ levels are elevated in prodromal and early disease stages. Obstruction of Aβ clearance through peripheral channels may ultimately result in excess accumulation in brain. Direct and indirect support for this possibility has been provided by several studies,[90,91] including an in vivo model in which hyperinsulinemia and insulin resistance were induced with high fat feeding in the Tg 2576 mouse model of AD, and were shown to increase brain Aβ levels.[63]

To summarize our model, as shown in Figure 7.3, peripheral insulin resistance and hyperinsulinemia lead to a depletion of brain insulin levels. As a result, intraneuronal Aβ release is inhibited and IDE levels are lowered,

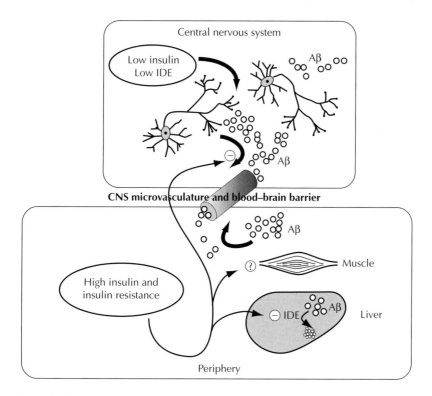

Figure 7.3

Model of peripheral hyperinsulinemia, insulin resistance, and Alzheimer's disease (AD) pathogenesis. IDE, insulin-degrading enzyme; Aβ, amyloid beta.

promoting intraneuronal Aβ accumulation and other negative effects of CNS insulin depletion. The accumulation of Aβ is compounded by obstruction of its clearance through the periphery. Peripheral hyperinsulinemia and insulin resistance reduce Aβ uptake and clearance in liver and other peripheral sites, causing a rise in peripheral Aβ levels. Plasma Aβ elevations interfere with clearance from brain to periphery, or enhance Aβ transport into brain.

IMPLICATIONS FOR TREATMENT

The preceding model suggests that restoring normal peripheral and brain insulin levels in persons with AD may improve cognition, and modulate Aβ. Any long-term treatment strategy in persons with AD must avoid significantly increasing insulin in the periphery. We have described two therapeutic options that fulfill this criterion: treatment with the insulin-sensitizing PPARγ (peroxisome proliferator-activated receptor gamma) agonist rosiglitazone, and selective supplementation of CNS insulin with an intranasal administration technique.

PPARγ agonists as insulin-sensitizing, anti-inflammatory agents

PPARγ is a ligand-activated nuclear transcription factor that lowers plasma insulin and free fatty acid (FFA) levels and improves insulin sensitivity. In the periphery, PPARγ is expressed highly in adipose tissue, where it plays a crucial role in adipogenesis, triglyceride storage, and regulation of FFA levels. Individuals with heterozygous loss of function mutations within the PPARγ ligand-binding domain have insulin resistance, early-onset T2DM, and dyslipidemia.[92] Thiazolidinediones, used clinically to treat T2DM, are potent synthetic PPARγ ligands. Their antidiabetic action is correlated with their PPARγ potency.[92] Given the greater expression of PPARγ in fat relative to skeletal muscle, changes in insulin sensitivity may reflect activity in adipocytes, where PPARγ activation:

1. increases fatty acid influx into adipocytes, thereby reducing fatty acid availability for muscles
2. decreases expression of tumor necrosis factor alpha (TNFα)
3. shifts fat from visceral to subcutaneous depots.[93]

Each of these actions can improve insulin sensitivity and reduce inflammation. Consistent with this notion, the thiazolidinedione rosiglitazone protects rats against acute inflammatory responses.[94] In humans with coronary artery disease, rosiglitazone reduces markers of endothelial cell activation and levels of acute-phase reactants such as C-reactive protein and fibrinogen.[95]

In brain, PPARγ has been detected in neurons and astrocytes,[96] where it influences cell survival, often through anti-inflammatory actions. In rats,

PPARγ agonists reduce inducible nitric oxide synthase (iNOS) expression and post-glutamate toxicity in cerebellar granule cells,[97,98] reduce lipopolysacharide-induced iNOS and cyclooxygenase-2 (COX-2) expression in cortical neurons[99] and glia,[100] and reduce microglial activation.[101] As noted, inflammation is a likely pathogenetic factor in AD. Amyloid plaques are associated with activated microglia and neurotoxic proinflammatory products,[102] and Aβ stimulates the secretion of neurotoxic proinflammatory products and activation of astrocytes. Interestingly, expression of PPARγ is increased in the temporal cortex of AD patients.[103] PPARγ agonists inhibit Aβ-stimulated monocyte differentiation into macrophages, activation of microglia, and Aβ-stimulated expression of cytokine genes and COX-2.[104] Thus, PPARγ activation may interfere with proinflammatory processes observed in AD. PPARγ effects on β-amyloid processing and deposition are more controversial. For example, it has been reported that proinflammatory cytokines stimulate the secretion of Aβ partially by increasing β-secretase activity, and that PPARγ activation inhibits proinflammatory effects on β-secretase activity and Aβ production.[105] Other investigators found minimal effects of PPARγ activation on reduction of Aβ burden associated with nonsteroidal anti-inflammatory drugs.[106,107] Finally, thiazolidinedione agonists increase glucose metabolism in astrocytes, although effects may not be mediated by PPARγ activation.[108] Since astrocytes provide energy substrates to neurons, increased astrocytic glucose metabolism may attenuate the effects of hypometabolism associated with AD. Thus, PPARγ agonists are promising therapeutic agents for AD for their demonstrated effects on insulin sensitivity, inflammation, and cerebral energy metabolism.

Intranasal pathways to the CNS

Intranasal insulin administration represents a second approach to restoring normal brain insulin levels in persons with AD. In the upper nasal cavity, olfactory sensory neurons are directly exposed, whereas their axons extend through the cribriform plate to the olfactory bulb. Following intranasal administration, drugs can be directly transported to the CNS, bypassing the periphery. Several extraneuronal and intraneuronal pathways from the nasal cavity to the CNS are possible. The extraneuronal pathways appear to rely on bulk flow transport through perineural channels to the brain or CSF. In a recent autoradiographic study, IGF-1, a peptide closely related to insulin, was administered intranasally to rats.[109] Within 30 minutes, IGF-1 signals traveled through channels connecting the nasal cavity with the olfactory bulb and rostral brain regions, with robust signals evident in hippocampus and amygdala. A second pathway was identified in channels associated with the peripheral trigeminal system that connects the nasal cavity with the brainstem and spinal cord. In a third extracellular pathway quick access to the CSF is obtained after absorption into the submucosa along the olfactory nerve and cribriform plate.[109–111] The CSF drains along the olfactory nerve and approaches the submucosa in the roof of the nasal cavity before reaching the nasal lymphatics. Large-molecular-weight molecules are commonly cleared from the CNS along this pathway into the deep cervical nodes, which receive afferent lymphatics from the nasal passages.[112,113] These extracellular pathways provide direct access to the CNS within minutes of intranasal administration.

Additionally, an intraneuronal pathway delivers drugs to the CNS hours or days later. Anterograde axoplasmic transport within olfactory sensory neurons has been demonstrated. For example, the lectin conjugate wheat germ agglutinin-horseradish peroxidase (WGA-HRP) delivered intranasally is endocytosed by olfactory neurons and transported to the olfactory bulbs and CNS within 6 hours in mice.[114–117]

Intranasal drug administration

Although there is a recent emphasis on the use of these pathways for drug delivery, their existence has been known for many years. Viruses and microorganisms,[118–120] metals,[121,122] dyes,[123,124] amino acids,[125] and proteins[117,126,127] have been shown to enter the CNS via nasal routes for decades. There are a variety of drugs that either cannot permeate the BBB to reach targets in the CNS, or which penetrate the BBB but can have harmful effects in the periphery. Recent investigations have defined drug characteristics that determine whether a specific agent can be transported to the CNS via intranasal routes. Substances with lower molecular weights are more likely to be transported to the CNS along intranasal pathways. A common approach to determining whether a specific drug can be transported to the CNS is measurement of the drug in CSF or brain following intranasal administration, while controlling or adjusting for drug transport to the periphery. Such research demonstrates that a significant number of therapeutic compounds are successfully delivered to the CNS following intranasal administration, including insulin,[110] neurotrophic factors,[128] antibiotics,[129] antivirals,[130] adrenergics,[131] antineoplastics,[132,133] estrogen and progesterone,[134,135] vasopressin,[136] cholecystokinin,[137] corticotropin-releasing hormone,[110] DNA plasmids,[138] and cocaine.[139].

Intranasal insulin effects in the CNS

Insulin, a peptide with a molecular weight of about 5800 kDa is delivered directly to the CNS following intranasal administration. Kern and colleagues[110] administered 40 IU of insulin intranasally in young, healthy adults. CSF and blood was sampled every 10–20 minutes for 80 minutes following administration. Insulin treatment resulted in increased CSF insulin levels within 10 minutes of administration compared with placebo with peak levels noted within 30 minutes. CSF insulin levels had not returned to baseline by the end of the 80-minute study. Blood glucose and insulin levels did not change, demonstrating that the effects in CSF are not due to transport from the nasal cavity to systemic circulation. This is consistent with a large literature that demonstrates insulin's poor transport from the nasal cavity into blood.[140] Although elevated CSF insulin levels do not conclusively demonstrate that brain insulin levels are similarly elevated, animal studies have shown significant drug uptake to brain regions such as the amygdala.[141]

Functional and cognitive studies of the acute and chronic effects of intranasal administration also support insulin's transport to the CNS. Sixty minutes of intranasal insulin treatment (20 IU every 15 minutes) induced changes in auditory-evoked brain potentials (AEPs) compared with placebo.[142] A recent study of the chronic effects of intranasal insulin treatment reported that 2 months of daily administration (4 × 40 IU/day) significantly improved verbal memory and enhanced mood in young healthy adults.[143] A second study of the chronic effects of intranasal insulin administration replicated declarative memory facilitation in healthy males, although details of this study are not published at this time.[144] Insulin treatment did not alter plasma glucose or insulin levels in either study. Additionally, we demonstrated that intranasal insulin acutely improves verbal memory in persons with AD without affecting plasma insulin or glucose levels[145] (Figure 7.4). These results also supported differences in insulin response related to presence or absence of the APOE-ε4 allele; in prior studies using intravenous insulin administration,

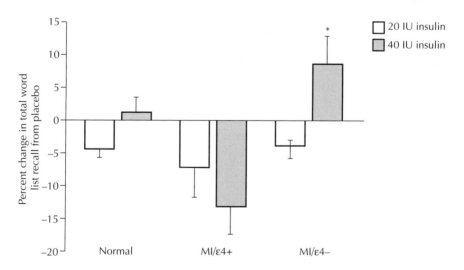

Figure 7.4

Effects of intranasal insulin treatment on verbal memory. Graph presents the percent change in total word list recall on the Buschke Selective Reminding Task compared with placebo in normal controls and memory-impaired (MI) subjects with and without the APOE-ε4 allele. Word list recall for MI subjects without the ε4 allele was significantly improved with 40 IU of insulin compared with saline treatment ($p=0.0323$). Word list recall for MI subjects with the ε4 allele was significantly lower with 40 IU of insulin compared with saline treatment ($p = 0.0044$).).

AD patients without the ε4 allele required higher doses of insulin to facilitate memory than did subjects with an APOE-ε4 allele.[19]

Increasing insulin levels in the CNS may have direct and indirect effects on insulin regulation in the periphery. Obesity, a condition closely linked to insulin resistance and diabetes, may represent an antecedent risk factor for AD.[146] Eight weeks of intranasal insulin administration (4 × 40 IU/day) decreased body fat and weight.[147] Thus, intranasal insulin administration may help regulate peripheral insulin levels that are often abnormally high in AD.

This novel approach to delivering insulin to the CNS has also been conducted with IGF-1. Insulin and IGF-1 are highly homologous, have similar receptor structure, bind to each other's receptors, and initiate the same signaling pathways.[148] Liu, Frey, and colleagues have shown that intranasal IGF-1 reduces infarct volume, reduces apoptosis, and improves neurologic function in rats with middle cerebral artery occlusion.[149–151] A recent report demonstrates that intranasal IGF-1 treatment is effective even when delayed for up to 6 hours after occlusion.[151] Together, these studies reinforce intranasal approaches to delivering insulin and related peptides to the CNS.

SUMMARY AND FUTURE DIRECTIONS

In this chapter, we have reviewed evidence that CNS insulin levels and activity are decreased for patients with AD. This decrement occurs in conjunction with peripheral hyperinsulinemia and insulin resistance. As a result, the normal activities of insulin in the brain, which influence memory, Aβ regulation, tau phosphorylation, neurotransmitter availability, and energy metabolism, are perturbed. Such perturbation may create a neurobiologic environment favoring AD pathogenesis.

This model supports the development of novel therapeutic approaches focused on augmenting or normalizing insulin levels without concomitantly raising peripheral insulin, through the use of insulin sensitizing agents such as the PPARγ agonists, or through intranasal insulin administration. Critical information is needed regarding the safety, feasibility, and potential efficacy of these novel approaches, which can be obtained in future large-scale clinical trials.

ACKNOWLEDGMENTS

Support for the studies described in this chapter was provided by the Department of Veterans Affairs, NIH (cite ADRC pilot 2, NIA AG-10880). Suzanne Craft is a consultant for GlaxoSmithKline, maker of rosiglitazone.

REFERENCES

1. Ritchie K, Lovestone S. The dementias. Lancet 2002; 360:1759–1766.

2. Banks WA, Jaspan JB, Huang W, Kastin AJ. Transport of insulin across the blood–brain barrier: saturability at euglycemic doses of insulin. Peptides 1997;18:1423–1429.

3. Baskin DG, Figlewicz DP, Woods SC, Porte D Jr, Dorsa DM. Insulin in the brain. Annu Rev Physiol 1987;49: 335–347.

4. Baura GD, Foster DM, Porte D Jr, et al. Saturable transport of insulin from plasma into the central nervous system of dogs in vivo. A mechanism for regulated insulin delivery to the brain. J Clin Invest 1993;92:1824–1830.

5. Giddings SJ, Chirgwin J, Permutt MA. Evaluation of rat insulin messenger RNA in pancreatic and extrapancreatic tissues. Diabetologia 1985;28:343–347.

6. Schechter R, Holtzclaw L, Sadiq F, Kahn A, Devaskar S. Insulin synthesis by isolated rabbit neurons. Endocrinology 1988;123:505–513.

7. Yalow RS, Eng J. Insulin in the central nervous system. Adv Metab Disord 1983;10:341–354.

8. Devaskar SU, Giddings SJ, Rajakumar PA, et al. Insulin gene expression and insulin synthesis in mammalian neuronal cells. J Biol Chem 1994;269: 8445–8454.

9. Singh BS, Rajakumar PA, Eves EM, et al. Insulin gene expression in immortalized rat hippocampal and pheochromocytoma-12 cell lines. Regul Pept 1997;69:7–14.

10 Abbott MA, Wells DG, Fallon JR. The insulin receptor tyrosine kinase substrate p58/53 and the insulin receptor are components of CNS synapses. J Neurosci 1999;19:7300–7308.

11. Baskin DG, Figlewicz DP, Woods SC, Porte D Jr, Dorsa DM. Insulin in the brain. Annu Rev Physiol 1987;49: 335–347.

12. Havrankova J, Roth J, Brownstein M. Insulin receptors are widely distributed in the central nervous system of the rat. Nature 1978;272:827–829.

13. Havrankova J, Schmechel D, Roth J, Brownstein M. Identification of insulin in rat brain. Proc Natl Acad Sci USA 1978;75:5737–5741.

14. Marks JL, Eastman CJ. Ontogeny of insulin binding in different regions of the rat brain. Dev Neurosci 1990;12:349–358.

15. Unger JW, Livingston JN, Moss AM. Insulin receptors in the central nervous system: localization, signalling mechanisms and functional aspects. Prog Neurobiol 1991;36:343–362.

16. Zhao W, Cavallaro S, Gusev P, Alkon DL. Nonreceptor tyrosine protein kinase pp60c-src in spatial learning: synapse-specific changes in its gene expression, tyrosine phosphorylation, and protein–protein interactions. Proc Natl Acad Sci USA 2000;97:8098–8103.

17. Craft S, Newcomer J, Kanne S, et al. Memory improvement following induced hyperinsulinemia in Alzheimer's disease. Neurobiol Aging 1996;17:123–130.

18. Craft S, Asthana S, Newcomer JW, et al. Enhancement of memory in Alzheimer disease with insulin and somatostatin, but not glucose. Arch Gen Psychiatry 1999; 56:1135–1140.

19. Craft S, Asthana S, Cook DG, et al. Insulin dose–response effects on memory and plasma amyloid precursor protein in Alzheimer's disease: interactions with apolipoprotein E genotype. Psychoneuroendocrinology 2003; 28:809–822.

20. Kern W, Peters A, Fruehwald-Schultes B, et al. Improving influence of insulin on cognitive functions in humans. Neuroendocrinology 2001;74:270–280.

21. Zhao W, Chen H, Xu H, et al. Brain insulin receptors and spatial memory.

Correlated changes in gene expression, tyrosine phosphorylation, and signaling molecules in the hippocampus of water maze trained rats. J Biol Chem 1999;274:34893–34902.

22. Schwartz MW, Figlewicz DF, Kahn SE, et al. Insulin binding to brain capillaries is reduced in genetically obese, hyperinsulinemic Zucker rats. Peptides 1990;11:467–472.

23. Wallum BJ, Taborsky GJ Jr, Porte D Jr, et al. Cerebrospinal fluid insulin levels increase during intravenous insulin infusions in man. J Clin Endocrinol Metab 1987;64:190–194.

24. Greenwood CE, Winocur G. Glucose treatment reduces memory deficits in young adult rats fed high-fat diets. Neurobiol Learn Mem 2001;75:179–189.

25. Vanhanen M, Koivisto K, Kuusisto J, et al. Cognitive function in an elderly population with persistent impaired glucose tolerance. Diabetes Care 1998;21:398–402.

26. Convit A, Wolf OT, Tarshish C, de Leon MJ. Reduced glucose tolerance is associated with poor memory performance and hippocampal atrophy among normal elderly. Proc Natl Acad Sci USA 2003;100:2019–2022.

27. Bingham EM, Hopkins D, Smith D, et al. The role of insulin in human brain glucose metabolism: an 18fluorodeoxyglucose positron emission tomography study. Diabetes 2002;51:3384–3390.

28. Reagan LP, Gorovits N, Hoskin EK, et al. Localization and regulation of GLUTx1 glucose transporter in the hippocampus of streptozotocin diabetic rats. Proc Natl Acad Sci USA 2001;98:2820–2825.

29. Schulingkamp RJ, Pagano TC, Hung D, Raffa RB. Insulin receptors and insulin action in the brain: review and clinical implications. Neurosci Biobehav Rev 2000;24:855–872.

30. Apelt J, Mehlhorn G, Schliebs R. Insulin-sensitive GLUT4 glucose transporters are colocalized with GLUT3-expressing cells and demonstrate a chemically distinct neuron-specific localization in rat brain. J Neurosci Res 1999;57:693–705.

31. Brant AM, Jess TJ, Milligan G, Brown CM, Gould GW. Immunological analysis of glucose transporters expressed in different regions of the rat brain and central nervous system. Biochem Biophys Res Commun 1993;192:1297–1302.

32. El Messari S, Leloup C, Quignon M, et al. Immunocytochemical localization of the insulin-responsive glucose transporter 4 (Glut4) in the rat central nervous system. J Comp Neurol 1998;399:492–512.

33. Livingstone C, Lyall H, Gould GW. Hypothalamic GLUT 4 expression: a glucose- and insulin-sensing mechanism? Mol Cell Endocrinol 1995;107:67–70.

34. Zhao WQ, Alkon DL. Role of insulin and insulin receptor in learning and memory. Mol Cell Endocrinol 2001;177:125–134.

35. Skeberdis VA, Lan J, Zheng X, Zukin RS, Bennett MV. Insulin promotes rapid delivery of N-methyl-D-aspartate receptors to the cell surface by exocytosis. Proc Natl Acad Sci USA 2001;98:3561–3566.

36. Ott A, Stolk RP, van Harskamp F, et al. Diabetes mellitus and the risk of dementia: The Rotterdam Study. Neurology 1999;53:1937–1942.

37. Peila R, Rodriguez BL, Launer LJ. Type 2 diabetes, APOE gene, and the risk for dementia and related pathologies: The Honolulu–Asia Aging Study. Diabetes 2002; 51:1256–1262.

38. Leibson CL, Rocca WA, Hanson VA, et al. The risk of dementia among persons with diabetes mellitus: a population-based cohort study. Ann N Y Acad Sci 1997;826:422–427.

39. Luchsinger JA, Tang MX, Shea S, Mayeux R. Hyperinsulinemia and risk of Alzheimer disease. Neurology 2004;63:1187–1192.

40. Kurochkin IV, Goto S. Alzheimer's beta-amyloid peptide specifically interacts with and is degraded by insulin degrading enzyme. FEBS Lett 1994;345:33–37.

41. Hoyer S. The aging brain. Changes in the neuronal insulin/insulin receptor signal transduction cascade trigger late-onset sporadic Alzheimer disease (SAD). A mini-review. J Neural Transm 2002;109:991–1002.

42. Frolich L, Blum-Degen D, Bernstein HG, et al. Brain insulin and insulin receptors in aging and sporadic Alzheimer's disease. J Neural Transm 1998;105:423–438.

43. Gasparini L, Gouras GK, Wang R, et al. Stimulation of beta-amyloid precursor protein trafficking by insulin reduces intraneuronal beta-amyloid and requires mitogen-activated protein kinase signaling. J Neurosci 2001;21:2561–2570.

44. Zhao L, Teter B, Morihara T, et al. Insulin-degrading enzyme as a downstream target of insulin receptor signaling cascade: implications for Alzheimer's disease intervention. J Neurosci 2004;24:11120–11126.

45. Authier F, Posner BI, Bergeron JJ. Insulin-degrading enzyme. Clin Invest Med 1996;19:149–160.

46. McDermott JR, Gibson AM. Degradation of Alzheimer's beta-amyloid protein by human and rat brain peptidases: involvement of insulin-degrading enzyme. Neurochem Res 1997;22:49–56.

47. Qiu W, Walsh D, Ye Z, et al. Insulin-degrading enzyme regulates extracellular levels of amyloid beta-protein by degradation. J Biol Chem 1998;273:32730–32738.

48. Sudoh S, Frosch MP, Wolf BA. Differential effects of proteases involved in intracellular degradation of amyloid β-protein between detergent-soluble and -insoluble pools in CHO-695 cells. Biochemistry 2002;41:1091–1099.

49. Abraham R, Myers A, Wavrant-DeVrieze F, et al. Substantial linkage disequilibrium across the insulin-degrading enzyme locus but no association with late-onset Alzheimer's disease. Hum Genet 2001;109:646–652.

50. Ait-Ghezala G, Abdullah L, Crescentini R, et al. Confirmation of association between D10S583 and Alzheimer's disease in a case–control sample. Neurosci Lett 2002;325:87–90.

51. Bertram L, Blacker D, Mullin K, et al. Evidence for genetic linkage of Alzheimer's disease to chromosome 10q. Science 2000;290:2302–2303.

52. Boussaha M, Hannequin D, Verpillat P, et al. Polymorphisms of insulin degrading enzyme gene are not associated with Alzheimer's disease. Neurosci Lett 2002;329:121–123.

53. Ertekin-Taner N, Graff-Radford N, Younkin LH, et al. Linkage of plasma Aβ42 to a quantitative locus on chromosome 10 in late-onset Alzheimer's disease pedigrees. Science 2000;290:2303–2304.

54. Myers A, Holmans P, Marshall H, et al. Susceptibility locus for Alzheimer's disease on chromosome 10. Science 2000;290:2304–2305.

55. Cook DG, Leverenz JB, McMillan PJ, et al. Reduced hippocampal insulin-degrading enzyme in late-onset Alzheimer's disease is associated with the apolipoprotein E-epsilon4 allele. Am J Pathol 2003;162:313–319.

56. Farris W, Mansourian S, Chang Y, et al. Insulin-degrading enzyme regulates the levels of insulin, amyloid beta-protein, and the beta-amyloid precursor protein intracellular domain in vivo. Proc Natl Acad Sci USA 2003;100:4162–4167.

57. Perez A, Morelli L, Cresto JC, Castano EM. Degradation of soluble amyloid beta-peptides 1–40, 1–42, and the Dutch variant 1–40Q by insulin degrading enzyme from Alzheimer

disease and control brains. Neurochem Res 2000;25:247–255.

58. Banks WA, Jaspan JB, Kastin AJ. Selective, physiological transport of insulin across the blood–brain barrier: novel demonstration by species-specific radioimmunoassays. Peptides 1997;18:1257–1262.

59. Schwartz MW, Figlewicz DF, Kahn SE, et al. Insulin binding to brain capillaries is reduced in genetically obese, hyperinsulinemic Zucker rats. Peptides 1990;11:467–472.

60. Gerozissis K, Orosco M, Rouch C, Nicolaidis S. Basal and hyperinsulinemia-induced immunoreactive hypothalamic insulin changes in lean and genetically obese Zucker rats revealed by microdialysis. Brain Res 1993; 611:258–263.

61. Kaiyala KJ, Prigeon RL, Kahn SE, Woods SC, Schwartz MW. Obesity induced by a high-fat diet is associated with reduced brain insulin transport in dogs. Diabetes 2000;49: 1525–1533.

62. Craft S, Peskind E, Schwartz MW, et al. Cerebrospinal fluid and plasma insulin levels in Alzheimer's disease: relationship to severity of dementia and apolipoprotein E genotype. Neurology 1998;50:164–168.

63. Ho L, Qin W, Pompl PN, et al. Diet-induced insulin resistance promotes amyloidosis in a transgenic mouse model of Alzheimer's disease. FASEB J 2004;18:902–904.

64. Giorgino F, Almahfouz A, Goodyear LJ, Smith RJ. Glucocorticoid regulation of insulin receptor and substrate IRS-1 tyrosine phosphorylation in rat skeletal muscle in vivo. J Clin Invest 1993;91:2020–2030.

65. Kupfer SR, Wilson EM, French FS. Androgen and glucocorticoid receptors interact with insulin degrading enzyme. J Biol Chem 1994;269: 20622–20628.

66. Ali M, Plas C. Glucocorticoid regulation of chloroquine nonsensitive insulin degradation in cultured fetal rat hepatocytes. J Biol Chem 1989; 264:20992–20997.

67. Harada S, Smith RM, Hu DQ, Jarett L. Dexamethasone inhibits insulin binding to insulin-degrading enzyme and cytosolic insulin-binding protein p82. Biochem Biophys Res Commun 1996;218:154–158.

68. Baura GD, Foster DM, Kaiyala K, et al. Insulin transport from plasma into the central nervous system is inhibited by dexamethasone in dogs. Diabetes 1996;45:86–90.

69. Kulstad JJ, McMillan PJ, Leverenz JB, et al. Effects of chronic glucocorticoid administration on insulin-degrading enzyme and amyloid-beta peptide in the aged macaque. J Neuropathol Exp Neurol 2005;64:139–146.

70. Davis KL, Davis BM, Greenwald BS, et al. Cortisol and Alzheimer's disease, I: Basal studies. Am J Psychiatry 1986;143:300–305.

71. Hartmann A, Veldhuis JD, Deuschle M, Standhardt H, Heuser I. Twenty-four hour cortisol release profiles in patients with Alzheimer's and Parkinson's disease compared to normal controls: ultradian secretory pulsatility and diurnal variation. Neurobiol Aging 1997;18:285–289.

72. Maeda K, Tanimoto K, Terada T, Shintani T, Kakigi T. Elevated urinary free cortisol in patients with dementia. Neurobiol Aging 1991;12:161–163.

73. Swanwick GR, Kirby M, Bruce I, et al. Hypothalamic–pituitary–adrenal axis dysfunction in Alzheimer's disease: lack of association between longitudinal and cross-sectional findings. Am J Psychiatry 1998;155:286–289.

74. Umegaki H, Ikari H, Nakahata H, et al. Plasma cortisol levels in elderly female subjects with Alzheimer's disease: a cross-sectional and longitudinal study. Brain Res 2000;881:241–243.

75. Peskind ER, Wilkinson CW, Petrie EC, Schellenberg GD, Raskind MA. Increased CSF cortisol in AD is a function of APOE genotype. Neurology 2001;56:1094–1098.

76. Touma C, Ambree O, Gortz N, et al. Age- and sex-dependent development of adrenocortical hyperactivity in a transgenic mouse model of Alzheimer's disease. Neurobiol Aging 2004;25:893–904.

77. Hong M, Lee V. Insulin and insulin-like growth factor-1 regulate tau phosphorylation in cultured human neurons. J Biol Chem 1997;272: 19547–19553.

78. Hanger DP, Hughes K, Woodgett JR, Brion JP, Anderton BH. Glycogen synthase kinase-3 induces Alzheimer's disease-like phosphorylation of tau: generation of paired helical filament epitopes and neuronal localisation of the kinase. Neurosci Lett 1992;147: 58–62.

79. Mandelkow EM, Drewes G, Biernat J, et al. Glycogen synthase kinase-3 and the Alzheimer-like state of microtubule-associated protein tau. FEBS Lett 1992;314:315–321.

80. Lovestone S, Reynolds CH, Latimer D, et al. Alzheimer's disease-like phosphorylation of the microtubule-associated protein tau by glycogen synthase kinase-3 in transfected mammalian cells. Curr Biol 1994;4:1077–1086.

81. Sperber BR, Leight S, Goedert M, Lee VM. Glycogen synthase kinase-3 beta phosphorylates tau protein at multiple sites in intact cells. Neurosci Lett 1995;197:149–153.

82. Schubert M, Gautam D, Surjo D, et al. Role for neuronal insulin resistance in neurodegenerative diseases. Proc Natl Acad Sci USA 2004;101:3100–3105.

83. Schubert M, Brazil DP, Burks DJ, et al. Insulin receptor substrate-2 deficiency impairs brain growth and promotes tau phosphorylation. J Neurosci 2003;23:7084–7092.

84. Craft S, Watson GS. Insulin and neurodegenerative disease: shared and specific mechanisms. Lancet Neurol 2004;3:169–178.

85. Gasparini L, Gouras GK, Wang R, et al. Stimulation of β-amyloid precursor protein trafficking by insulin reduces intraneuronal β-amyloid and required mitogen-activated protein kinase signaling. Journal of Neuroscience 2001;21:2561–2570.

86. Carro E, Trejo JL, Gomez-Isla T, LeRoith D, Torres-Aleman I. Serum insulin-like growth factor I regulates brain amyloid-beta levels. Nat Med 2002;8:1390–1397.

87. Hone E, Martins IJ, Fonte J, Martins RN. Apolipoprotein E influences amyloid-beta clearance from the murine periphery. J Alzheimers Dis 2003;5:1–8.

88. Kulstad JJ, Cook DG, Craft S. Modulation of amyloid-beta degradation in hepatic (hepG2) cells by insulin. Soc Neurosci Abstr 2003; 29.

89. Mayeux R, Honig LS, Tang MX, et al. Plasma A[beta]40 and A[beta]42 and Alzheimer's disease: relation to age, mortality, and risk. Neurology 2003; 61:1185–1190.

90. Li L, Cao D, Garber DW, Kim H, Fukuchi K. Association of aortic atherosclerosis with cerebral beta-amyloidosis and learning deficits in a mouse model of Alzheimer's disease. Am J Pathol 2003;163:2155–2164.

91. Shie FS, LeBoeur RC, Jin LW. Early intraneuronal Abeta deposition in the hippocampus of APP transgenic mice. Neuroreport 2003;14:123–129.

92. Gurnell M. PPARgamma and metabolism: insights from the study of human genetic variants. Clin Endocrinol (Oxf) 2003 59:267–277.

93. Ferre P. The biology of peroxisome proliferator-activated receptors: relationship with lipid metabolism and insulin sensitivity. Diabetes 2004; 53(Suppl 1):S43–S50.

94. Cuzzocrea S, Pisano B, Dugo L, et al. Rosiglitazone, a ligand of the peroxisome proliferator-activated receptor-gamma, reduces acute inflammation. Eur J Pharmacol 2004;483:79–93.

95. Sidhu JS, Cowan D, Kaski JC. The effects of rosiglitazone, a peroxisome proliferator-activated receptor-gamma

agonist, on markers of endothelial cell activation, C-reactive protein, and fibrinogen levels in non-diabetic coronary artery disease patients. J Am Coll Cardiol 2003;42:1757–1763.

96. Moreno S, Farioli-Vecchioli S, Ceru MP. Immunolocalization of peroxisome proliferator-activated receptors and retinoid X receptors in the adult rat CNS. Neuroscience 2004;123: 131–145.

97. Heneka MT, Klockgether T, Feinstein DL. Peroxisome proliferator-activated receptor-gamma ligands reduce neuronal inducible nitric oxide synthase expression and cell death in vivo. J Neurosci 2000;20:6862–6867.

98. Uryu S, Harada J, Hisamoto M, Oda T. Troglitazone inhibits both postglutamate neurotoxicity and low-potassium-induced apoptosis in cerebellar granule neurons. Brain Res 2002;924:229–236.

99. Kim EJ, Kwon KJ, Park JY, et al. Effects of peroxisome proliferator-activated receptor agonists on LPS-induced neuronal death in mixed cortical neurons: associated with iNOS and COX-2. Brain Res 2002; 941:1–10.

100. Kitamura Y, Kakimura J, Matsuoka Y, et al. Activators of peroxisome proliferator-activated receptor-gamma (PPARgamma) inhibit inducible nitric oxide synthase expression but increase heme oxygenase-1 expression in rat glial cells. Neurosci Lett 1999;262:129–132.

101. Bernardo A, Ajmone-Cat MA, Levi G, Minghetti L. 15-deoxy-delta12,14-prostaglandin J2 regulates the functional state and the survival of microglial cells through multiple molecular mechanisms. J Neurochem 2003;87:742–751.

102. Landreth GE, Heneka MT. Anti-inflammatory actions of peroxisome proliferator-activated receptor gamma agonists in Alzheimer's disease. Neurobiol Aging 2001;22:937–944.

103. Kitamura Y, Shimohama S, Koike H, et al. Increased expression of cyclooxygenases and peroxisome proliferator-activated receptor-gamma in Alzheimer's disease brains. Biochem Biophys Res Commun 1999;254:582–586.

104. Combs CK, Johnson DE, Karlo JC, Cannady SB, Landreth GE. Inflammatory mechanisms in Alzheimer's disease: inhibition of beta-amyloid-stimulated proinflammatory responses and neurotoxicity by PPARgamma agonists. J Neurosci 2000;20:558–567.

105. Sastre M, Dewachter I, Landreth GE, et al. Nonsteroidal anti-inflammatory drugs and peroxisome proliferator-activated receptor-gamma agonists modulate immunostimulated processing of amyloid precursor protein through regulation of beta-secretase. J Neurosci 2003;23:9796–9804.

106. Sagi SA, Weggen S, Eriksen J, Golde TE, Koo EH. The non-cyclooxygenase targets of non-steroidal anti-inflammatory drugs, lipoxygenases, peroxisome proliferator-activated receptor, inhibitor of kappa B kinase, and NF kappa B, do not reduce amyloid beta 42 production. J Biol Chem 2003;278:31825–31830.

107. Yan Q, Zhang J, Liu H, et al. Anti-inflammatory drug therapy alters beta-amyloid processing and deposition in an animal model of Alzheimer's disease. J Neurosci 2003;23:7504–7509.

108. Dello Russo C, Gavrilyuk V, Weinberg G, et al. Peroxisome proliferator-activated receptor gamma thiazolidinedione agonists increase glucose metabolism in astrocytes. J Biol Chem 2003; 278:5828–5836.

109. Thorne RG, Pronk GJ, Padmanabhan V, Frey WH 2nd. Delivery of insulin-like growth factor-I to the rat brain and spinal cord along olfactory and trigeminal pathways following intranasal administration. Neuroscience 2004;127:481–496.

110. Born J, Lange T, Kern W, et al. Sniffing neuropeptides: a transnasal approach to the human brain. Nat Neurosci 2002;5:514–516.

111. Frey WH, 2nd. Intranasal delivery: bypassing the blood–brain barrier to deliver therapeutic agents to the brain and spinal cord. Drug Deliv Technol 2002;2:46–49.

112. Bradbury MWB, Cserr HF. Drainage of cerebral interstitial fluid and of cerebrospinal fluid into lymphatics. In: Johnson MG, ed. Experimental Biology of the Lymphatic Circulation. New York: Elsevier, 1985: 355–394.

113. Weller RO. Pathology of cerebrospinal fluid and interstitial fluid of the CNS: significance for Alzheimer disease, prion disorders and multiple sclerosis. J Neuropathol Exp Neurol 1998; 57:885–894.

114. Baker H, Spencer RF. Transneuronal transport of peroxidase-conjugated wheat germ agglutinin (WGA-HRP) from the olfactory epithelium to the brain of the adult rat. Exp Brain Res 1986;63:461–473.

115. Balin BJ, Broadwell RD, Salcman M, el-Kalliny M. Avenues for entry of peripherally administered protein to the central nervous system in mouse, rat, and squirrel monkey. J Comp Neurol 1986;251:260–280.

116. Broadwell RD, Balin BJ. Endocytic and exocytic pathways of the neuronal secretory process and trans-synaptic transfer of wheat germ agglutinin-horseradish peroxidase in vivo. J Comp Neurol 1985;242:632–650.

117. Shipley MT. Transport of molecules from nose to brain: transneuronal anterograde and retrograde labeling in the rat olfactory system by wheat germ agglutinin-horseradish peroxidase applied to the nasal epithelium. Brain Res Bull 1985;15:129–142.

118. Bodian D, Howe HA. Experimental studies on intraneuronal spread of poliomyelitis virus. Bull Johns Hopkins Hosp 1941;68:248–267.

119. Faber HK. The early lesions of poliomyelitis after intranasal inoculation. J Pediatr 1938;13:10–37.

120. Fairbrother RW, Hurst EW. The pathogenesis of, and propagation of the virus in, experimental poliomyelitis. J Pathol Bact 1930;33:17–45.

121. Czerniawska A. Experimental investigations on the penetration of ^{198}Au from nasal mucous membrane into cerebrospinal fluid. Acta Otolaryngol 1970;70:58–61.

122. Gopinath PG, Gopinath G, Kumar TCA. Target site of intranasally sprayed substances and their transport across the nasal mucosa: a new insight into the intranasal route of drug delivery. Curr Ther Res 1978;23:596–607.

123. Clark WE, Gros L. Anatomical investigation into the routes by which infections may pass from the nasal cavities into the brain. Ministry of Health Report on Public Health and Medical Subjects. Vol. 54. London: HM Stationary Office, 1929.

124. Faber WM. The nasal mucosa and the subarachnoid space. Am J Anat 1937;62:121–148.

125. Weiss P, Holland Y. Neuronal dynamics and axonal flow, II. The olfactory nerve as a model test object. Proc Natl Acad Sci USA 1967;57:258–264.

126. Kristensson K, Olsson Y. Uptake of exogenous proteins in mouse olfactory cells. Acta Neuropathol (Berl) 1971;19:145–154.

127. Thorne RG, Emory CR, Ala TA, Frey WH, 2nd. Quantitative analysis of the olfactory pathway for drug delivery to the brain. Brain Res 1995;692: 278–282.

128. Thorne RG, Frey WH 2nd. Delivery of neurotrophic factors to the central nervous system: pharmacokinetic considerations. Clin Pharmacokinet 2001;40:907–946.

129. Sakane T, Akizuki M, Yoshida M, et al. Transport of cephalexin to the cerebrospinal fluid directly from the nasal

cavity. J Pharm Pharmacol 1991;43: 449–451.

130. Seki T, Sato N, Hasegawa T, Kawaguchi T, Juni K. Nasal absorption of zidovudine and its transport to cerebrospinal fluid in rats. Biol Pharm Bull 1994;17:1135–1137.

131. Anand Kumar TC, David GFX, Kumar K, Umberkoman B, Krishnamoorthy MS. A new approach to fertility regulation by interfering with neuroendocrine pathways. In: Anand Kumar TC, ed. Proceedings of International Symposium on Neuroendocrine Regulation of Fertility: Basel: Karger, 1976:314–322.

132. Wang F, Jiang X, Lu W. Profiles of methotrexate in blood and CSF following intranasal and intravenous administration to rats. Int J Pharm 2003;263:1–7.

133. Wang F, Jiang X, Lu W. Intranasal delivery of methotrexate to the brain in rats bypassing the blood–brain barrier. Drug Deliv Technol 2004; 4:48–55.

134. Anand Kumar TC, David GFX, Umberkoman B, Saini KD. Uptake of radioactivity by body fluids and tissues in rhesus monkeys after intravenous injection or intranasal spray of tritium-labeled estradiol and progesterone. Curr Sci 1974;43:435–439.

135. Anand Kumar TC, David GF, Sankaranarayanan A, Puri V, Sundram KR. Pharmacokinetics of progesterone after its administration to ovariectomized rhesus monkeys by injection, infusion, or nasal spraying. Proc Natl Acad Sci USA 1982;79:4185–4189.

136. Pietrowsky R, Struben C, Molle M, Fehm HL, Born J. Brain potential changes after intranasal vs. intravenous administration of vasopressin: evidence for a direct nose–brain pathway for peptide effects in humans. Biol Psychiatry 1996;39:332–340.

137. Pietrowsky R, Thiemann A, Kern W, Fehm HL, Born J. A nose–brain pathway for psychotropic peptides: evidence from a brain evoked potential study with cholecystokinin. Psychoneuroendocrinology 1996;21:559–572.

138. Oh YK, Kim JP, Hwang TS, et al. Nasal absorption and biodistribution of plasmid DNA: an alternative route of DNA vaccine delivery. Vaccine 2001;19:4519–4525.

139. Chow HS, Chen Z, Matsuura GT. Direct transport of cocaine from the nasal cavity to the brain following intranasal cocaine administration in rats. J Pharm Sci 1999;88:754–758.

140. Illum L. Nasal drug delivery: new developments and strategies. Drug Discov Today 2002;7:1184–1189.

141. Chen XQ, Fawcett JR, Rahman YE, Ala TA, Frey IW. Delivery of nerve growth factor to the brain via the olfactory pathway. J Alzheimers Dis 1998;1:35–44.

142. Kern W, Born J, Schreiber H, Fehm HL. Central nervous system effects of intranasally administered insulin during euglycemia in men. Diabetes 1999;48:557–563.

143. Benedict C, Hallschmid M, Hatke A, et al. Intranasal insulin improves memory in humans. Psychoneuroendocrinology 2004;29:1326–1334.

144. Stockhorst U, de Fries D, Steingrueber HJ, Scherbaum WA. Insulin and the CNS: effects on food intake, memory, and endocrine parameters and the role of intranasal insulin administration in humans. Physiol Behav 2004;83: 47–54.

145. Reger MA, Watson GS, Frey II WH, et al. Effects of intranasal insulin on cognition in memory-impaired older adults: modulation by APOE genotype. Neurobiol Aging 2005;25 (Suppl 2):S35–42.

146. Gustafson D, Rothenberg E, Blennow K, Steen B, Skoog I. An 18-year follow-up of overweight and risk of Alzheimer disease. Arch Intern Med 2003;163:1524–1528.

147. Hallschmid M, Benedict C, Schultes B, et al. Intranasal insulin reduces body fat in men but not in women. Diabetes 2004;53:3024–3029.

148. Pandini G, Frasca F, Mineo R, et al. Insulin/insulin-like growth factor I hybrid receptors have different biological characteristics depending on the insulin receptor isoform involved. J Biol Chem 2002;277:39684–39695.

149. Liu XF, Fawcett JR, Thorne RG, DeFor TA, Frey WH 2nd. Intranasal administration of insulin-like growth factor-I bypasses the blood–brain barrier and protects against focal cerebral ischemic damage. J Neurol Sci 2001;187:91–97.

150. Liu XF, Fawcett JR, Thorne RG, Frey WH 2nd. Non-invasive intranasal insulin-like growth factor-I reduces infarct volume and improves neurologic function in rats following middle cerebral artery occlusion. Neurosci Lett 2001;308:91–94.

151. Liu XF, Fawcett JR, Hanson LR, Frey WH. The window of opportunity for treatment of focal cerebral ischemic damage with noninvasive intranasal insulin-like growth factor-I in rats. J Stroke Cerebrovasc Dis 2004;13: 16–23.

8
Atypical antipsychotics in dementia

Lesley M Blake and Jacobo Mintzer

INTRODUCTION

Alzheimer's disease is a complex disorder characterized by both cognitive and behavioral alterations, including symptoms of psychosis such as delusions and hallucinations.[1] The prevalence of psychosis in Alzheimer's disease varies among studies, but it is generally thought to be between 30 and 60%.[2–6] The consequence of the presence of psychotic symptoms in these patients is severe, causing added stress to the patient, as well as adding to the burden of the disease for family and caregivers.[7] Patients with psychosis of Alzheimer's disease are also more likely to have disruptive aggressive behaviors, further adding to caregiver burden,[8] and decreasing quality of life.

Patients with psychosis of Alzheimer's disease tend to have more severe cognitive and functional deficits compared to those with Alzheimer's disease without psychosis who were matched for other clinical characteristics.[9–11] Psychotic symptoms have been associated with a more rapid decline in cognition and function,[4,12,13] and are a predictor of early long-term care placement.[14,15] The following is a brief summary of the key issues to be considered when evaluating and considering treatment for patients suffering from psychosis of Alzheimer's disease.

PSYCHOTIC SYMPTOMS IN ALZHEIMER'S DISEASE

The mechanism leading to psychosis in patients with Alzheimer's disease is unknown, but clear differences exist between psychosis of Alzheimer's disease and other types of psychotic disorders such as schizophrenia.[16] Specifically, the hallucinations in psychosis of Alzheimer's disease tend to be visual rather than auditory, whereas the reverse is true in schizophrenia. Schneiderian first-rank symptoms (such as voices commenting on a patient's behavior) are very rare in Alzheimer's disease. The delusions experienced by patients with Alzheimer's disease are typically paranoid, simple, and non-bizarre compared to those of schizophrenic patients, which tend to be complex and more bizarre. In Alzheimer's disease, psychotic symptoms tend to be more prominent in the middle phase of the illness, and may persist for several years.[13,17] However, they may disappear in the more advanced stages of the illness. This could be related to actual diminution of symptoms or may be related to the fact that patients with severe dementia may not be able to articulate or act on their hallucinations and delusions.

The *Diagnostic and Statistical Manual of Mental Disorders*, 4th edn (DSM-IV)[18] describes criteria for the diagnoses of the dementing illnesses, and recommends additional coding if delusions are a prominent feature of the illness, but does not define criteria as such for this subcategory. Jeste and Finkel[19] proposed criteria to aid in the diagnosis of psychosis of Alzheimer's disease as a distinct syndrome. These criteria may apply to the psychotic symptoms associated with other dementias, such as vascular dementia or dementia with Lewy bodies. They also help distinguish the psychotic symptoms of Alzheimer's disease from those of other causes, such as delirium or drug-induced psychotic symptoms in Parkinson's disease.

Although the mood stabilizers valproate and carbamazepine could be useful in managing the behavioral symptoms of dementia,[20,21] antipsychotic medications are recommended as a first-line treatment for the management of the behavioral disorders of Alzheimer's disease.[22] The use of conventional antipsychotics has been limited due to concerns over their side-effect profiles, including risk of sedation, hypotension, anticholinergic effects, and both short-term and long-term extrapyramidal side effects. Concerns about the potential risks of using these medications in the elderly nursing home population was one of the factors leading up to the passage of the nursing home reform provisions of the Omnibus Budget Reconciliation Act of 1987.

The newer antipsychotic agents, combined serotonin (5-hydroxytryptamine, 5-HT) and dopamine agents, appear to have a more benign side-effect profile, but still need to be used with caution in the elderly cognitively impaired population. Elderly patients with dementia are at particular risk for drug-related adverse events. Physiologic changes of aging affect both the pharmacokinetics and pharmacodynamics of drugs.[23] Changes occur in the absorption, distribution, metabolism, and elimination of medications, resulting from the physiologic changes in gastrointestinal mobility, hepatic blood flow, and renal function, as well as the changes in the composition of lean and fat body mass. There also are alterations in neurotransmitters and receptor sensitivity, which can alter the magnitude of drug effects, and increase the risk of adverse events.

EFFICACY AND SAFETY OF ATYPICAL ANTIPSYCHOTICS IN DEMENTIA

There are currently six atypical antipsychotic medications which are approved for use in the United States: clozapine, risperidone, olanzapine, quetiapine, aripiprazole, and ziprasidone. None of these medications are currently approved by the Food and Drug Administration (FDA) for use in patients with behavioral disorders of dementia, but approval for some drugs in the treatment of psychosis of Alzheimer's disease could come as soon as early 2005. The following is a review of the available information on the use of atypical antipsychotics in dementia.

Clozapine

The prototypical atypical antipsychotic drug is clozapine. Clozapine exhibits a modest dopamine (D_2) receptor blockade, a somewhat greater serotonin (5-HT_2) receptor blockade, and a pronounced cholinergic muscarinic (M_1) receptor blockade. It tends to be highly sedating, very anticholinergic, and potentially cardiotoxic. It can significantly lower the seizure threshold, and may produce leukopenia,[24] requiring close monitoring of complete blood counts. There are no published placebo-controlled, randomized studies of clozapine in the treatment of behavioral disturbances of dementia such as psychosis. One small retrospective study which focused on patients with dementia[25] found that there was an improvement in irritability and social interest, and no leukopenia was reported. However, 4 of the 18 patients discontinued clozapine due to delirium, somnolence, and restlessness. Another study[26] showed improvement in hallucinations and delusions. Clozapine may have a use for controlling treatment-resistant psychotic symptoms in patients with dementia, or in those with severe tardive dyskinesia or extrapyramidal symptoms, but its side-effect profile precludes its use as a first-line drug.

The recommended starting dose of clozapine is 6.25–12.5 mg/day, with increases of no more than 6.25–12.5 mg once or twice a week. Maintenance doses should generally be 50–100 mg/day.[27]

Risperidone

Risperidone has a higher affinity for 5-HT_2 than D_2 receptors, but lacks affinity for muscarinic receptors. It is the most studied atypical antipsychotic in the treatment of elderly patients with dementia. The efficacy in the treatment of psychosis of Alzheimer's disease has been evaluated in case series, open studies, and large, multicenter, placebo-controlled studies. Early case studies[28,29] of elderly patients with dementia indicated that risperidone therapy reduced delusions, aggression, and agitation in these patients, and improved participation in social activities, without producing severe extrapyramidal symptoms.

Further case series and open-label, retrospective, and pharmacoepidemiologic studies also suggested that risperidone is effective for the control of agitation and aggression in patients with dementia.[30–35] The results of these studies are summarized in Table 8.1.

The efficacy of risperidone (0.5–2.0 mg/day) in treating psychosis and aggression in elderly patients with dementia was also studied in 4 large, multicenter, double-blind, placebo-controlled studies.[36–39] The first, and largest study, was done in US long-term care facilities.[36] A total of 625 patients were treated with fixed doses of risperidone (0.5, 1.0, or 2.0 mg/day) or placebo for

Table 8.1	Uncontrolled studies of Risperdal (risperidone) in the management of behavior disorders of dementia		
Study	Design	n	Dose
Brennan et al[30]	Case series	8	1.0–2.0 mg/day
Frenchman and Prince[31]	Retrospective chart review	60	1.0 mg/day (median)
Frenchman[32]	Retrospective chart review	65	1.1 mg/day (mean)
Gareri et al[33]	Open-label trial	13	1.0 or 2.0 mg/day
Goldberg and Goldberg[34]	Open-label trial	109	0.25 to >1.0 mg/day
Zarate et al[35]	Retrospective chart review	122	1.6 mg/day (mean)

Outcome
Decrease in agitation according to clinical impression
Improvement in target symptoms in 94% of patients
Improvement in behavioral symptoms in 85% of patients
Significant decrease in NPI at endpoint
Clinical impression of improvement in 81% of patients
Improvement in CGI in 85.2% of patients

NPI, Neuropsychiatric Inventory, CGI, Clinical Global Impression.

12 weeks. At endpoint, the patients who had received 1.0 or 2.0 mg/day of risperidone had a significantly greater improvement in scores on the Behavioral Pathology in Alzheimer's Disease (BEHAVE-AD)[40] rating scale total score and the psychosis and aggressive subscales than did those patients on placebo. Significant improvements were seen on all of the paranoid/delusional ideation items of the psychosis subscale. Improvement was seen as early as the second week of treatment. Similar improvement was found in the Cohen-Mansfield Agitation Inventory (CMAI)[41] aggression scores.

The second study was undertaken in Europe and looked at the effects of 12 weeks of active treatment with flexible doses (0.5–4.0 mg/day) of risperidone, haloperidol, or placebo on aggression and agitation in 344 elderly patients with dementia.[37] The mean dose at endpoint was 1.1 mg/day of risperidone, and 1.2 mg/day of haloperidol. Reductions in the BEHAVE-AD total score were significantly greater with risperidone than with placebo at week 12. Aggression cluster scores for the BEHAVE-AD and CMAI were significantly lower for the patients on risperidone than those on placebo at endpoint and week 12. There was also a significantly greater reduction in the BEHAVE-AD aggression score with risperidone than haloperidol at week 12.

In the third study,[38] which was done in Australia and New Zealand, 345 elderly patients with dementia and behavioral disorders, residing in long-term care, were randomized to receive either a flexible dose of risperidone (mean dose 0.95 mg/day) or placebo. Outcome measures included the CMAI and the BEHAVE-AD. There was a significant reduction in the CMAI total aggression score for the patients receiving risperidone compared with those on placebo. A similar improvement was seen in the CMAI non-aggression subscale, and for the BEHAVE-AD total and psychotic subscale.

A further nursing home study, carried out in the United States, enrolled 473 patients with dementia and behavior disorders.[39] The patients were assigned to either flexible dose risperidone (mean dose 1.03 mg/day) or placebo for an 8-week treatment period. Both groups improved significantly on the BEHAVE-AD psychotic subscale; however, no statistically significant difference between risperidone and placebo was observed. In a protocol-specified analysis among patients with more advanced dementia, Mini-Mental State Examination (MMSE) 5 to 9, there was a statistical trend for improvement on the BEHAVE-AD psychosis subscale for risperidone over placebo. The results of these studies are summarized in Table 8.2.

There also are data indicating that risperidone may be effective in the treatment of other behavioral disturbances of dementia such as alterations in the sleep–wake cycle. A post-marketing surveillance study[42] was done involving 4499 patients with behavioral and psychotic symptoms of dementia. In this study, the patient's sleep–wake cycle was rated by their physicians on a 4-point scale, where 0 denoted no sleep disturbance, and 4 denoted very severe sleep disturbance. At baseline, the mean score was 2.3, indicating moderate-to-severe sleep disturbance, and after 8 weeks of treatment with risperidone at a mean dosage of 1.6 mg/day, the mean score was 1.0. This was a statistically significant improvement from moderate–severe disturbance to mild disturbance. It was suggested that the D_2 antagonism of risperidone improved dementia-related disruption of circadian rhythms, and that the $5\text{-}HT_{2A}$ antagonism improved sleep structure.

Despite the concerns about the possibility of frequent and severe adverse events occurring in elderly patients, clinical studies have reported that

Table 8.1	Double-blind placebo-controlled trials of risperidone for the management of the behavioral disorders of dementia		
Study	n	Design	Dose
Katz et al[36]	625	0.5, 1.0, 2.0 mg/day	12 weeks
DeDeyn et al[37]	344	1.1 mg/day (mean)	12 weeks
Brodaty et al[38]	345	0.95 mg/day (mean)	12 weeks
Mintzer et al[39]	473	1.03 mg/day (mean)	8 weeks

Outcome
Significant improvement in BEHAVE-AD and CMAI compared to placebo
Significant improvement in BEHAVE-AD and CMAI (aggression) compared to placebo
Significant improvement in BEHAVE-AD and CMAI compared to placebo
Significant improvement in BEHAVE-AD (psychosis) in patients on risperidone and placebo

BEHAVE-AD, Behavioral Pathology in Alzheimer's Disease; CMAI, Cohen-Mansfield Agitation Inventory.

risperidone was well tolerated during the trials.[31,32,35,36,43,44] and was better tolerated than conventional antipsychotics.[37,44]

Several studies have reported a low rate of extrapyramidal side effects in elderly patients being treated with risperidone.[31,32,36,37,43-45] A 1 year open-label study of 330 patients with dementia who were treated with risperidone (mean modal dose 0.96 mg/day) showed a cumulative incidence of new-onset tardive dyskinesia of 2.6%, and a decrease in dyskinesia severity among patients who had dyskinesia at baseline.[45] Another study where patients received risperidone (mean dose 3.7 mg/day) showed a rate of tardive dyskinesia of 4.3% at 12 months, a rate much lower than the expected rate of 26.0% with conventional antipsychotics.[43]

In a double-blind study of patients with dementia, where the patients were receiving 0.5–2.0 mg/day of risperidone, no cases of tardive dyskinesia were noted.[36] Furthermore, among patients receiving 0.5 and 1.0 mg/day, there were no differences in extrapyramidal side effect ratings between these patients and those patients on placebo. Similarly, in a 12-week double-blind study in patients with dementia,[37] the rate of extrapyramidal symptoms (EPS) in the risperidone group did not differ significantly from that in the placebo group.

In a 12-week open-label trial of risperidone in elderly patients with psychotic disorders[44] there was a transient increase in the Extrapyramidal Symptom Rating Scale (ESRS) scores, but this was followed by a decrease in scores, such that there was a significant decrease in scores from baseline at the endpoint. Studies comparing risperidone and haloperidol have shown a lower incidence of tardive dyskinesia at 9 months;[45] significantly lower ESRS scores at 3 months,[37] and a lower incidence of extrapyramidal side effects among elderly patients treated with risperidone.[31]

Risperidone has a low muscarinic receptor-binding affinity,[46] and the low incidence of clinically significant anticholinergic side effects seen with risperidone in the elderly is consistent with this.[35-37,43,44] Several studies have reported some sedation in elderly patients receiving risperidone,[35-37,40] but the incidence was low, and it seemed to be a dose-related and time-limited effect. Sedation has been reported to be associated with a rapid increase in risperidone dosing, and may be less of a problem during longer-term therapy.[47] One study (with a mean dose of 2.4 mg/day) reported that 15% of patients had some somnolence,[44] and another study, with a mean risperidone dose of 1.1 mg/day, reported that somnolence occurred in 12.2% of patients.[37] In the fixed-dose study,[36] patients who received 0.5, 1.0, and 2.0 mg/day of risperidone had a reported incidence of somnolence of 10.1%, 16.9%, and 27.9%, respectively. Finally, a low incidence of sedation (3.3%) was seen among patients receiving a mean risperidone dose of 1.6 mg/day.[39]

Falls are common in nursing home residents, and falls associated with medication use are a frequent cause of hospital admission.[48] In a post-hoc analysis of a large double-blind trial of patients with dementia,[49] there was a significant reduction in fall rates among patients treated with risperidone 1.0 mg/day compared with placebo. In another large double-blind study, the incidence of falls among patients with dementia who received risperidone was no different from that of patients receiving placebo.[37] Orthostatic hypotension has been related to falls,[24] and is of particular concern in the elderly. In risperidone studies, orthostasis occurred in fewer than 10% of patients,[35–37,43,44] and many patients were on concomitant antihypertensive medications.[35]

In some trials conducted in patients with dementia, a higher incidence of cerebrovascular adverse events (CAEs) was noted to occur with risperidone than with placebo. There was no relationship between dosage of risperidone and the incidence of CAEs, but the majority of patients experiencing CAEs had one or more pre-existing risk factors for cerebrovascular events, including prior history of stroke, atrial fibrillation, and hypertension.[50] A retrospective cohort study[51] evaluated the relative risk of stroke with risperidone use in the elderly with dementia, compared to olanzapine, haloperidol, benzodiazepines, and acetylcholinesterase inhibitors. The authors concluded that risperidone does not pose a greater risk for stroke-related events than treatment with the other medications. Further information related to this safety issue is anticipated as more data become available.

Some adverse events that are of concern in younger patients using antipsychotics do not seem to be as relevant in the elderly. Risperidone has not been reported to cause significant weight gain in the elderly.[43] Although risperidone may increase prolactin levels, no significant clinical correlation between prolactin levels and adverse events has been noted.[52]

Olanzapine

Olanzapine produces moderate blockade of D_2, $5HT_2$, and M_1 receptors. Its half-life is about 30 hours, and it can be dosed once a day, preferably at bedtime. Its most frequent side effects include sedation, postural hypotension, anticholinergic reactions, and weight gain. A placebo-controlled, flexible-dose study in 238 outpatients, which included patients with dementia complicated by psychosis or agitation, showed no benefit with olanzapine therapy.[53] However, the primary objective of the study was to evaluate the tolerability of olanzapine relative to dose, and low doses (mean dose 2.7 mg/day) were used. Olanzapine was subsequently found to show benefit in doses of 5 and 10 mg/day in a 6-week, double-blind, placebo-controlled study of 206 nursing home residents with Alzheimer's disease and behavioral disturbances.[54] The study examined the efficacy and tolerability of fixed doses of olanzapine (5, 10, or 15 mg/day). The proportion of patients showing a 50% or greater decline in the Neuropsychiatric Inventory (NPI)[55] was significantly more for patients on 5 and 10 mg/day of olanzapine than for patients on placebo or 15 mg/day of olanzapine. Furthermore, the patients on 5 and 10 mg/day of olanzapine showed a significant improvement in the sum of the agitation/aggression, hallucinations, and delusional items of the NPI, compared with placebo.

Adverse events seen in this study included pain, accidental injury, somnolence, and abnormal gait. Somnolence and abnormal gait were the only adverse events that had a significantly higher incidence in the olanzapine group than in the placebo group and were dose-related effects. There was a significantly higher rate of adverse events that could be related to anticholinergic side effects in the 15 mg/day olanzapine group than in the placebo group. The frequency of EPS was no greater in the olanzapine group than in the placebo group.

Nineteen patients in this study who were randomized to olanzapine met the criteria for dementia with Lewy bodies. There was a reduction in psychotic symptoms in those patients on 5 and 10 mg/day, but not on 15 mg/day of olanzapine.[56] There was no increase in Parkinsonism noted. In an open trial of olanzapine in 8 patients diagnosed with dementia with Lewy bodies, doses of 2.5–7.5 mg/day were prescribed. Two patients showed clear improvement, 3 patients had minimal improvement, and 3 patients could not tolerate the drug due to worsening cognition and extrapyramidal side effects even on the lowest doses.[57]

The suggested initial dose of olanzapine in patients with dementia is 1–5 mg/day (average 2.5 mg/day), with a maintenance dose of 5–15 mg/day.[27]

Quetiapine

Quetiapine is a dibenzothiazepine derivative with a higher affinity for $5-HT_2$ receptors than D_2 receptors. It inhibits histaminic (H_1) and α_1-adrenergic receptors but has minimal affinity for muscarinic receptors. It is largely protein bound and is metabolized by cytochrome 34A to inactive metabolites. Its half-life is approximately 7 hours, and twice a day dosing is usual.

In an open trial of quetiapine in 151 older patients with psychosis, approximately half of whom had Alzheimer's disease, the most common side effects were dizziness, sedation, postural hypotension, and agitation.[58] EPS occurred in 6% of patients, and included akathisia, tremor, and nuchal rigidity. The dose range of quetiapine was 25–800 mg/day, with a median dose of 100 mg/day. There was at least a 20% reduction from baseline in total scores on the Brief Psychiatric Rating Scale (BPRS),[59] in 52% of all subjects.

Data from a subset of 78 patients diagnosed with Alzheimer's disease from this study were retrospectively analyzed. The effect of quetiapine on hostility in patients with psychosis related to Alzheimer's disease was evaluated using the BPRS factor V score (mean of hostility, suspiciousness, uncooperativeness, excitement), the BPRS hostility item, and a BPRS hostility cluster score (mean of anxiety, tension, hostility, suspiciousness, uncooperativeness, excitement). Significant improvement in hostility was seen during the 52 weeks of the study. The median quetiapine dose was 100 mg/day.[60]

A 10-week double-blind placebo-controlled trial compared the efficacy and safety of quetiapine, haloperidol, and placebo in 284 nursing home residents with Alzheimer's dementia. Doses of quetiapine ranged from 25–600 mg/day, and of haloperidol from 0.5 to 12 mg/day. No difference was seen on measures of psychosis across the 3 treatments, whereas both antipsychotics significantly improved the BPRS agitation factor compared with placebo.[61] Patients in the quetiapine group had statistically significantly better functional status, as assessed by the Multidimensional Observation Scale for Elderly Subjects (MOSES), Physical Self-Maintenance Scale (PMS), and BPRS anergia factor, and fewer extrapyramidal side effects or anticholinergic adverse events compared with the haloperidol group. Clinically relevant adverse events included somnolence, postural hypotension, dizziness, weight gain, and weight loss in all groups. Fewer patients in the quetiapine group experienced accidental injuries than patients treated with haloperidol or placebo. The incidence of falls was similar between treatment groups.

A further 10-week, fixed-dose, multicenter, double-blind, placebo-controlled study of quetiapine in 333 nursing home patients with agitation associated with dementia compared the efficacy and tolerability of quetiapine at the doses of either 100 or 200 mg/day with placebo.[62] Improvement in the Positive and Negative Syndrome Scale – Excitement Component (PANSS-EC) and Clinical Global Impression (CGI) was seen in the 200 mg/day group compared with the placebo group (significant in the observed case analysis; nearly significant in the last observation carried forward analysis). The incidence of adverse reactions was similar in all treatment groups, except for somnolence, which was more common in the quetiapine groups. The ESRS was low, and similar in all treatment groups.

A post-hoc analysis was performed on data from 260 patients in the above study who were diagnosed with Alzheimer's disease.[63] Treatment with 200 mg/day of quetiapine resulted in a significantly greater reduction in PANSS-EC and in CGIC (Clinical Global Impression of Change) scores compared with placebo (on both the observed cases and last observations carried forward analyses). The incidence of adverse events was comparable among treatment groups. No CAEs were reported in any group during treatment. The incidence rates of postural hypotension and falls were similar among groups, and the rate of somnolence was low with quetiapine and was not a dose-related effect.

A 5-week open, comparative study of quetiapine (25–125 mg/day) or haloperidol (0.5–4 mg/day) was undertaken in 28 patients with a diagnosis of Alzheimer's disease and behavioral disorders. Both quetiapine and haloperidol reduced delusions and agitation, as measured by the NPI. Compared to haloperidol, quetiapine improved depression, anxiety, and aberrant motor behavior. Actimetry was used to monitor circadian rest–activity cycles. Patients on quetiapine had quieter, more consolidated sleep.[64]

A recent double-blind, placebo-controlled, 26-week three-arm study compared quetiapine to the cholinesterase inhibitor rivastigmine or placebo in patients with Alzheimer's disease and agitation.[65] The target dose of rivastigmine was 3–6 mg twice daily and the target dose for quetiapine was 25–50 mg twice daily. No difference was observed in any of the treatment arms for agitation and neither of the two interventions was superior to placebo. Patients who had scores greater than 10 on the Severe Impairment Battery[66] were assessed with this instrument at 6 and 26 weeks. Patients on rivastigmine had a 3.1 point decline, patients on quetiapine exhibited an 11.3 point decline, whereas patients on placebo had a 3.3-point improvement (week 26). The authors concluded that quetiapine may exacerbate cognitive deficits in patients with Alzheimer's disease. The expected decline on the Severe Impairment Battery in 26 weeks in untreated patients is 10–20 points,[66] within the range observed in those on quetiapine. Patients on rivastigmine had less marked decline, as expected for a cholinesterase inhibitor-type cognitive enhancing agent. The unexpected improvement in the placebo group remains unexplained. The target dose for quetiapine was probably too low, as demonstrated in other recent clinical trials. The study is important in demonstrating that lower doses of quetiapine are insufficient to produce an anti-agitation response.

The recommended starting dose of quetiapine in elderly patients is between 100 and 200 mg, with the optimal target dose being 200 mg/day.[27] According to one study, quetiapine can be safely titrated up to 200 mg in 8 days, increasing the dose in 25 mg intervals on a daily basis.

Aripiprazole

Aripiprazole is a potent partial agonist at D_2 dopamine receptors, putatively acting as a functional antagonist at D_2 receptors in a hyperdopaminergic environment and a functional agonist at D_2 receptors in a hypodopaminergic environment. It is a serotonin antagonist at $5-HT_{2A}$ and a partial agonist at $5-HT_{1A}$ receptors. It has a moderate affinity for alpha$_1$-adrenergic and histamine (H_1) receptors and no appreciable affinity for cholinergic muscarinic receptors.[67]

The efficacy and safety of aripiprazole in patients with Alzheimer's disease and psychosis was evaluated through a 10-week placebo-controlled study of 208 outpatients. The patients received placebo or 2–15 mg/day of aripiprazole on a flexible dosing schedule.

There was a significant difference in the decrease of BPRS core and psychosis subscale scores in the aripiprazole group compared with the placebo group, and a non-significant decrease in the NPI psychosis subscale score.[66] Aripiprazole was well tolerated in general; the most common adverse events reported were urinary tract infection (8% vs 12% placebo), accidental injury (8% vs 5%), somnolence (8% vs 1%), bronchitis (6% vs 3%), and extrapyramidal side effects (5% vs 4%).

A second 10-week placebo-controlled trial involved 256 nursing home or assisted living facility residents. Patients randomized to aripiprazole received flexible doses of 2–15 mg/day, with a mean dose at endpoint of 8.6 mg. Symptoms of psychosis, evaluated by the NPI-NH (Neuropsychiatric Inventory – Nuring Home Version) psychosis subscale, improved in both the aripiprazole and placebo groups, but there was no statistically significant difference between groups. Aripiprazole treatment resulted in significant improvement in the total NPI-NH and BPRS scores compared with placebo. The incidence of adverse events was similar in the two groups, with somnolence being the only adverse event showing a greater than 10% difference in incidence between the two groups. EPS-related events were reported in 4% of patients on placebo, and 5% on aripiprazole.[69]

The starting dose of aripiprazole in the elderly patient with dementia is from 2 to 10 mg/day, with a target dose of up to 30 mg/day.

Ziprasidone

Ziprasidone has a higher affinity for 5-HT$_2$ receptors than for D$_2$ receptors and minimal anticholinergic effects.[70] There is a greater degree of Qtc prolongation than with the other newer agents,[71] and the drug is contraindicated in persons with a Qtc interval longer than 500 ms, and in combination with other drugs that prolong Qtc or inhibit the metabolism of ziprasidone. A case series of 10 patients with behavioral disturbances related to dementia who were treated with ziprasidone showed marked clinical improvement in their mean NPI scores.[72] There are currently double-blind, placebo-controlled studies under way that are looking at the efficacy and safety of ziprasidone in patients with dementia, but none are published as of now.

ATYPICAL ANTIPSYCHOTICS AS A TREATMENT CLASS OF AGENTS IN DEMENTIA

To date, most researchers and clinicians agree that atypical antipsychotic agents such as clozapine, risperidone, olanzapine, quetiapine, and aripiprazole are useful in treating patients with behavioral syndromes of dementia, including psychosis and agitation of Alzheimer's disease. There are no definitive guidelines to aid the clinicians in the choice of the specific agent to be used. Most available data show all studied agents to have a modest but reliable beneficial effect. Issues that need to be considered when prescribing such compounds include comorbid medical illnesses, concurrent medications, and past experience with medications.

Safety of these classes of compounds is an important consideration. Metabolic abnormalities have been reported with the use of atypical antipsychotics. The American Diabetes Association, the American Psychiatric Association, the American Association of Clinical Endocrinologists, and the North American Association for the Study of Obesity published a consensus paper on this issue.[73] Using the available evidence, the panel observed that clozapine and olanzapine, which produce the greatest weight gain, are also associated with the greatest increase in total cholesterol, low-density lipoprotein (LDL) cholesterol, and triglycerides, and with decreased high-density lipoprotein (HDL) cholesterol. Risperidone and quetiapine appear to have intermediate effects on lipids, whereas the risk of diabetes is unclear. Some studies show a greater risk – others do not. Aripiprazole and ziprasidone have limited data, but the available clinical trials do not show a greater risk of obesity, hyperlipidemia, or diabetes. There is very little evidence about the absolute or relative risk of metabolic effects of these agents in the elderly patients with dementia.

Concern about CAEs with atypical antipsychotics in patients with dementia has led to warnings about an increase in adverse events with risperidone, olanzapine, and aripiprazole. It is difficult to fully evaluate the risk in this population, which already has a high rate of medical comorbidity leading to an increased vulnerability to CAEs. Thus, it is prudent to prescribe these agents only when the risks of untreated symptoms and the benefits of medications outweigh the potential risks of adverse events, including CAEs.

The issue of limited data directly comparing atypical antipsychotics in patients with dementia has been addressed in a 36-week, National Institute of Mental Health-sponsored study, comparing risperidone, olanzapine, quetiapine, citalopram, and placebo as treatment for patients with Alzheimer's disease with delusions, hallucinations, and/or agitation.[74] The early results of this trial have shown that risperidone, olanzapine, and quetiapine were tolerated and effective in this population,[75] and further results which should be available soon, may help guide the clinician to find the most effective psychotropic treatment for dementia associated with hallucinations, delusions, and agitation.

The diagnostic categorization of the behavioral disturbances of dementia is an ongoing process. The development of diagnostic criteria for psychosis of Alzheimer's disease[19] is a step in this direction, and current efforts are underway to get FDA approval for atypical antipsychotics for treatment of this condition. Much more research into the long-term benefits and risks of atypical antipsychotics is needed, but, together with non-pharmacologic approaches and caregiver support, the atypical antipsychotics play an important role in the management of behavioral and psychological symptoms associated with dementia.

CONCLUSION

There is no universally accepted treatment for the different behavioral syndromes commonly seen in patients with dementia. Behavioral interventions remain the first-line treatment for these patients. Atypical antipsychotics provide a small, but reliable beneficial effect in the treatment of behavioral symptoms, especially agitation and psychosis, in Alzheimer's disease. These compounds appear to have a relatively benign side-effect profile; however, there is a risk of extrapyramidal side effects, somnolence, and orthostatic hypotension, and possibly an increased risk for CAEs. They remain a useful tool in the management of the patient with behavioral disorders of dementia.

REFERENCES

1. Alzheimer A, Stelzmann RA, Schnitzlein HN, Murtagh FR. An English translation of Alzheimer's 1907 paper, ;Uber eine eigenartige Erkankung der Hirnrinde'. Clin Anat 1995;8(6):429–431.

2. Wragg RE, Jeste DV. Overview of depression and psychosis in Alzheimer's disease. Am J Psychiatry 1989;146:577–587.

3. Sweet RA, Hamilton RL, Lopez OL, et al. Psychotic symptoms in Alzheimer's disease are not associated with more severe neuropathologic features. Int Psychogeriatr 2000;12: 547–558.

4. Paulsen JS, Salmon DP, Thal I, et al. Incidence of and risk factors for hallucinations and delusions in patients with probable Alzheimer's disease. Neurology 2000;54:1965–1971.

5. Mendez M, Martin R, Smyth KA, et al. Psychiatric symptoms associated with Alzheimer's disease. J Neuropsychiatry Clin Neurosci 1990;2: 28–33.

6. Forstl H, Burns A, Levy R, et al. Neuropathological correlates of psychotic phenomena in confirmed Alzheimer's disease. Br J Psychiatry 1994;165:53–59.

7. Kaufer DI, Cummings JL, Christine D, et al. Assessing the impact of neuropsychiatric symptoms in Alzheimer's disease: the Neuropsychiatric Inventory Caregiver Distress Scale. J Am Geriatr Soc 1998;46(2):210–215.

8. Aarsland D, Cummings JL, Yenner G, Miller B. Relationship of aggressive behavior to other neuropsychiatric symptoms in patients with Alzheimer's disease. Am J Psychiatry 1996:153(2):243–247.

9. Jeste DV, Wragg RE, Salmon DP, et al. Cognitive deficits of patients with and without delusions. Am J Psychiatry 1992:149(2):184–189.

10. Paulsen JS, Ready RE, Stout JC, et al. Neurobehaviors and psychotic symptoms in Alzheimer's disease. J Int Neuropsychol Soc 2000;6(7): 815–820.

11. Stern Y, Mayeux R, Sano M, et al. Predictors of disease course in patients with probable Alzheimer's disease. Neurology 1987;37(10): 1649–1653.

12. Drevets WC, Rubin EH. Psychotic symptoms and the longitudinal course of senile dementia of the Alzheimer type. Biol Psychiatry 1989;25(1):39–48.

13. Levy ML, Cummings JL, Fairbanks LA, et al. Longitudinal assessment of symptoms of depression, agitation, and psychosis in 181 patients with Alzheimer's disease. Am J Psychiatry 1996;153(11);1438–1443.

14. Magni E, Binetti G, Bianchetti A, Trabucchi M. Risk of mortality and institutionalization in demented patients with delusions. J Geriatr Psychiatry Neurol 1996;9(3): 123–126.

15. Lopez OL, Wisniewski SR, Becker JT, et al. Psychiatric medication and abnormal behavior as predictors of progression in probable Alzheimer's disease. Arch Neurol 1999;56(10): 1266–1272.

16. Jeste DV, Heaton SC, Paulsen JS, et al. Clinical and neuropsychological comparison of psychotic depression with nonpsychotic depression and schizophrenia. Am J Psychiatry 1996; 153(4):490–496.

17. Devanand DP, Jacobs DM, Tang MX, et al. The course of psychopathologic features in mild to moderate Alzheimer's disease. Arch Gen Psychiatry 1997;54:257–263.

18. Diagnostic and Statistical Manual of Mental Disorders, 4th edn, text revision. Washington DC: American Psychiatric Publishing, 2000.

19. Jeste DV, Finkel SI. Psychosis of Alzheimer's disease and related dementias. Diagnostic criteria for a distinct syndrome. Am J Geriatr Psychiatry 2000;8:29–34.

20. Mellow AM, Solano-Lopez C, Davis S. Sodium valproate in the treatment of behavioral disturbance in dementia. J Geriatr Psychiatry Neurol 1993;6:205–209.

21. Tariot PN, Erb R, Leibovici A, et al. Carbamazepine treatment of agitation in nursing home patients with dementia: a preliminary study. J Am Geriatr Soc 1994;42:1160–1166.

22. American Psychiatric Association Work Group on Alzheimer's Disease and Related Dementias. Practice guidelines for the treatment of patients with Alzheimer's disease and other dementias of late life. Am J Psychiatry 1997;154(Suppl 5):1–39.

23. Catterson ML, Preskorn SH, Martin RL. Pharmacodynamic and pharmacokinetic considerations in geriatric psychopharmacology. Psychiatr Clin North Am 1997;20:205–218.

24. Finkel S. Pharmacology of antipsychotics in the elderly: a focus on atypicals. J Am Geriatr Soc 2004; 52(12):S258–265.

25. Oberholzer AF, Hendriksen C, Monsch AU, et al. Safety and effectiveness of low dose clozapine in psychogeriatric patients: a preliminary study. Int Psychogeriatr 1992;4: 187–195.

26. Salzman C, Vaccaro B, Lieff J, et al. Clozapine in older patients with psychosis and behavioral disruption. Am J Geriatr Psychiatry 1995;3:26–33.

27. Jeste DV, Rockwell E, Harris J, et al. Conventional vs. newer antipsychotics in elderly patients. Am J Geriatr Psychiatry 1999;7:70–76.

28. Madhusoodanan S, Brenner R, Araujo L, et al. Efficacy of Risperidone treatment for psychoses associated with schizophrenia, schizoaffective disorder, bipolar disorder or senile dementia in 11 geriatric patients: a case series. J Clin Psychiatry 1995;56: 514–518.

29. Jeanblanc W, Davis YB. Risperidone for treating associated related aggression. Am J Psychiatry 1995;152:1239.

30. Brennan R, Lonergan V, Quilinan T, et al. Case studies on the use of risperidone for the treatment of agitation of elderly patients with dementia. J Drug assessment: 1999;2.247–253.

31. Frenchman IB, Prince T. Clinical experience with risperidone, haloperidol, and thioridazine for dementia-associated behavioral disturbance. Int Psychogeriatr 1997; 9:431–445.

32. Frenchman IB. Risperidone, haloperidol, and olanzapine for the treatment of behavioral disturbances in nursing home patients: a retrospective analysis. Curr Ther Res Clin Exp 2000;61:742–750.

33. Gareri P, Cotroneo A, Marchiso U, et al. Risperidone in the treatment of behavioral disorders of elderly patients with dementia. Arch Gerontol Geriatr 2001;33(Suppl 7):173–182.

34. Goldberg RJ, Goldberg J. Risperidone for dementia-related disturbed behavior in nursing home residents: a clinical experience. Int Psychogeriatr 1997;9:65–68.

35. Zarate CA Jr, Baldessarini RJ, Siegal AJ, et al. Risperidone in the elderly: a pharmacoepidemiologic study. J Clin Psychiatry 1997;58:311–317.

36. Katz IR, Jeste DV, Mintzer JE, et al. Comparison of risperidone and placebo for psychosis and behavioral disturbances associated with dementia: a randomized, double blind trial. J Clin Psychiatry 1999;60:107–115.

37. DeDeyn PP, Rabheru K, Rasmussen A, et al. A randomized trial of risperidone, placebo, and haloperidol for behavioral symptoms of dementia. Neurology 1999;53:946–955.

38. Brodaty H, Ames D, Snowdon J, et al. A randomized placebo-controlled trial of risperidone for the treatment

of aggression, agitation, and psychosis of dementia. J Clin Psychiatry 2003;64:134–143.

39. Mintzer J, Weiner M, Greenspan A, et al. Efficacy and safety of a flexible dose of risperidone versus placebo in the treatment of psychosis of Alzheimer's disease. Presented at the International College of Geriatric Psychoneuropharmacology, October 14–17, 2004, Basel, Switzerland.

40. Reisberg B, Borenstein J, Salob SP, et al. Behavioral symptoms in Alzheimer's disease: phenomenology and treatment. J Clin Psychiatry 1987; 48(5 Suppl):9–15.

41. Cohen-Mansfield J, Marx MS, Rosenthal AS. A description of agitation in a nursing home. J Gerontol 1989;44:M77–M84.

42. Schwalen S. Risperidone: effects on sleep-wake cycle disturbances in dementia. Presented at the 10th Congress of the International Psychogeriatric Association; September 9–14, 2001; Nice, France.

43. Davidson M, Harvey PD, Vervarcke J, et al. A long-term, multicenter, open label study of risperidone in elderly patients with psychosis. Int J Geriatr Psychiatry 2000;15:506–514.

44. Maadhusoodanan S, Brecher M, Brenner R, et al. Risperidone in the treatment of elderly patients with psychotic disorders. Am J Geriatr Psychiatry 1999;7:132–138.

45. Jeste DV, Okamoto A, Napolitano J, et al. Low incidence of persistent tardive dyskinesia in elderly patients with dementia treated with risperidone. Am J Psychiatry 2000;157:1150–1155.

46. Richelson E. Receptor pharmacology of neuroleptics: relation to clinical effects. J Clin Psychiatry 1999;60 (Suppl 10):5–14.

47. Conley RR. Risperidone side effects. J Clin Psychiatry 2000;61(Suppl 8):20–23.

48. Cooper JW. Adverse drug reaction-related hospitalizations of nursing facility patients: a 4-year study. South Med J 1999;92:485–490.

49. Katz IR, Schneider L, Kozma C, et al. Risk of falls in dementia patients: analysis of a randomized, double blind risperidone trial. Presented at Second Annual Meeting. International Congress of Psychoneuropharmacology, October 10–12, 2002, Barcelona, Spain.

50. Greenspan A, Eerdekens M, Mahmoud R. Is there an increased rate of cerebrovascular adverse events, including mortality, among dementia patients treated with risperidone? Presented at the International College of Geriatric Psychopharmacology, San Juan, Puerto Rico, December 14, 2003.

51. Kozma C, Engelhart L, Long S, et al. Absence of increased relative stroke risk in elderly dementia patients treated with risperidone versus other antipsychotics (poster). Presented at the International College of Geriatric Psychopharmacology, San Juan, Puerto Rico; December 13, 2003.

52. Kleinberg DL, Davis JM, de Coster R, et al. Prolactin levels and adverse events in patients treated with risperidone. J Clin Psychopharmacol 1999;19:57–61.

53. Satterlee WG, Reams SG, Burns PR, et al. A clinical update on olanzapine treatment in schizophrenia and in elderly Alzheimer's disease patients. Psychopharmacol Bull 1995; 31:534.

54. Street JS, Clark WS, Gannon KS, et al. Olanzapine treatment of psychotic and behavioral symptoms in patients with Alzheimer's disease in nursing care facilities: a double-blind, randomized, placebo-controlled trial. The HGEU Study Group. Arch Gen Psychiatry 2000;57:968–976.

55. Cummings JL, Mega M, Gray K, et al. The Neuropsychiatric Inventory: comprehensive assessment of psychopathology in dementia. Neurology 1994; 44:2308-2314.

56. Cummings JL, Street J, Masterman D, Clark WS. Efficacy of olanzapine in the treatment of psychosis in dementia with Lewy bodies. Dement Geriatr Cogn Disord 2002;13(2):67–73.

57. Walker A, Grace J, Overshot R, et al. Olanzapine in dementia with Lewy bodies: a clinical study. Int J Geriatr Psychiatry 1999;14:459–466.

58. McManus DQ, Arvantis LA, Kowalcyk BB. Quetiapine, a novel antipsychotic: experience in elderly patients with psychotic disorders. J Clin Psychiatry 1999; 60:292–298.

59. Overall JE, Gorham DR. The Brief Psychiatric Rating Scale (BPRS): recent developments in ascertainment and scaling. Psychopharmacol Bull 1988;24:97–98.

60. Schneider L, Yeung P, Sweitzer D, et al. Effects of Seoquel (quetiapine) on reducing hostility and psychosis in patients with Alzheimer's disease (poster). Presented at 152nd annual meeting of the American Psychiatric Association, May 15–20, 1999, Washington, DC.

61. Tariot P, Schneider L, Katz I, et al. Quetiapine in nursing home residents with Alzheimer's dementia and psychosis (poster). Presented at the 15th annual meeting of the American Association for Geriatric Psychiatry, February 24–27, 2002, Orlando, FL.

62. Zhong K, Tariot P, Minkwitz MC, et al. Quetiapine for the treatment of agitation in elderly institutionalized patients with dementia: a randomized, double blind trial (poster). Presented at the 9th International Conference on Alzheimer's Disease and Related Disorders, July 17–22, 2004, Philadelphia, PA.

63. Zhong K, Tariot P, Minkwitz M, et al. Quetiapine treatment of behavioral disturbance in patients with Alzheimer's disease (poster). Presented at the 18th annual meeting of the American Association for Geriatric Psychiatry, March 3–6, 2005, San Diego, CA.

64. Savaskan E, Schnitzler C, Schroder C, et al. Quetiapine improves behavioural, psychological and sleep-wake disturbances in patients with Alzheimer's disease (poster). Presented at the 12th Congress of the Association of European Psychiatrists, April 14–18, 2004, Geneva, Switzerland.

65. Ballard C, Margallo-Lana M, Juszczak E, et al. Quetiapine and rivastigmine and cognitive decline in Alzheimer's disease: randomised double blind placebo controlled trial. BMJ 2005; doi: 10.1136/bmj.38369.459988.8F.

66. Schmitt FA, Ashford W, Ernesto C, et al. The Severe Impairment Battery: concurrent validity and the assessment of longitudinal change in Alzheimer's disease. Alzheimer Dis Assoc Disord 1997;11:S51–S56.

67. Burris KD, Molski TF, Xu C, et al. Aripiprazole, a novel antipsychotic, is a high-affinity partial agonist at human dopamine D2 receptors. J Pharmacol Exp Ther. 2002:302: 381–389.

68. De Deyn PP, Jeste D, Mintzer J. Aripirazole in dementia of the Alzheimer's type (poster). Presented at the 16th annual meeting of the American Association for Geriatric Psychiatry, March 1–4, 2003, Honolulu, HI.

69. Streim JE, McQuade RD, Stock E, et al. Aripiprazole treatment of institutionalized patients with psychosis of Alzheimer's dementia (poster). Presented at the 17th annual meeting of the American Association for Geriatric Psychiatry, February 24–27, 2004, Baltimore, MD.

70. Schmidt AW, Lebel LA, Howard HR, et al. Ziprasidone: a novel antipsychotic agent with a unique human binding profile. Eur J Pharmacol 2001;425:197–201.

71. Gury C, Canceil O, Iaria P. [Antipsychotic drugs and cardiovascular safety: current studies of prolonged QT interval and risk of ventricular arrhythmia.] Encephale 2000;26:62–72. [in French].

72. Berkowitz A. Ziprasidone for elderly dementia: case series (poster). Presented at the 156th annual meeting of the American Psychiatric Association, May 17–23, 2003, San Francisco, CA.

73. American Diabetes Association, American Psychiatric Association. Consensus Development Conference on Antipsychotic Drugs and Obesity and Diabetes. Diabetes Care 2004;27: 596–601.

74. Schneider LS, Ismail MS, Dagerman K, et al. Clinical Antipsychotic Trials of Intervention Effectiveness (CATIE): Alzheimer's disease trial. Schizophr Bull 2003;29:57–72.

75. Schneider LS, Tariot P, Ismail MS, et al. Clinical Antipsychotic Trials of Intervention Effectiveness: Alzheimer's Disease (CATIE-AD): First Outcomes Report. (Poster) Presented at the 18th annual meeting of the American Association for Geriatric Psychiatry, March 3–6, 2005, San Diego, CA.

9

Treatment of vascular risk factors to delay Alzheimer's disease?

Frank-Erik de Leeuw, Raj Kalaria, and Philip Scheltens

INTRODUCTION

The potential link between vascular disease and Alzheimer's disease (AD) has gained considerable importance in recent years. There appears good evidence from epidemiologic studies to suggest that vascular factors, including a history of hypertension in mid life, high cholesterol, diabetes type 2 and hyperhomocysteinemia, increase the risk of succumbing to cognitive dysfunction and acquiring AD. Although risk may be reduced by treatment and management of vascular disease prior to onset of cognitive impairment, there is a lack of robust support for use of various agents to decrease incidence or impede progression to AD from the various large trials conducted thus far. The use of antihypertensives may be the best recommended, although with the caution that, in AD patients, blood pressure (BP) may already be low.

BACKGROUND

There is an increasing body of evidence that vascular factors such as history of hypertension, high cholesterol, hyperhomocysteinemia, and diabetes increase the risk of acquiring AD. There are, however, very few data on the treatment of vascular risk in AD patients with the purpose of improving cognition or impeding progression of decline other than preventing new vascular events. The fact that treatment of vascular risk factors, and especially hypertension, has a dramatic impact on the incidence of AD (in patients with pre-existent vascular disease such as isolated systolic hypertension, but *without* pre-existing cognitive dysfunction) does not necessarily imply a beneficial effect of this treatment in patients *with* pre-existing cognitive dysfunction or even dementia. This chapter addresses this particular topic, based on a review of existing published information, and provides a short historical introduction to highlight the fact that vascular factors had been previously considered but were forgotten for a long period of time until their rediscovery in recent years. We also summarize findings on treatment effects of BP-lowering drugs, statins, glucose, and homocysteine-lowering drugs on the course of AD.

The notion of an association between vascular risk factors and dementia was mentioned more than 100 years ago. At that time, it was thought most of the dementias were caused by hardening of the arteries, causing slow strangulation of blood flow to the brain. The term 'arteriosclerotic dementia' was introduced. Alois Alzheimer and Emil Kraepelin, who put Alzheimer's name to a dementia syndrome in the young patient they described, were also aware that prevalent dementias in those days (at the beginning of the 20th century) most frequently occurred in persons over 60–70 years old. It was for this latter reason perhaps, and the neuropathologic similarities between the dementias, that Alzheimer's disease came to be applied to both young and older demented people. Thus, vascular causes of AD were realized in those early days; however, they are now being reinvestigated because of advances in recognition of different treatable components of vascular disease and its link with cognitive function.[1]

BLOOD PRESSURE

Blood pressure is possibly the risk factor most studied in this context. Given the association of increased BP levels with ischemic brain lesions, it is likely that increased BP contributes to the development of more subtle cerebral processes that result from small vessel disease,[2,3] and lead to cognitive impairment and dementia.[4] However, the evidence for this is far from clear. In a large review from over 10 studies, including older normotensive and hypertensive persons, Seux and Forette[5] found that in four of these studies there was no relation between systolic or diastolic BP and cognition or dementia at all and, in one study, a positive correlation between both systolic and diastolic BP and cognition was evident. Nevertheless, the majority of the studies showed a clear negative association between BP and cognition, indicating that higher BP was associated with lower cognition. These studies also delineate that concurrent examination of BP and cognition is conceptually wrong, since BP changes in earlier life, rather than concurrent BP, may reflect the actual brain damage. This pitfall has been illustrated in a study by Skoog,[6] and later confirmed by other researchers.[7,8] In the Gothenburg H-70 study, a longitudinal population-based study of 70 year olds, repeated measurements on BP were available, prior to the diagnosis of dementia. It appeared that those who developed dementia at age 79–85 years old had a higher BP at age 70 years old compared with those who did not. But, even more remarkable, was their finding of decreased BP in the years preceding onset of AD. This was even more evident in those AD patients with white matter lesions, as seen on computed tomography (CT). Therefore, concurrent scrutiny of BP and cognition may obscure true associations, especially if the process of cognitive decline has already begun.

A more appropriate approach could be to investigate the relationship between BP and cognition longitudinally, in which BP is measured years before the cognitive assessments. Such an approach was implemented in the Framingham Study, with its decades of follow-up on people not treated for BP.[9] The study confirmed that those with the highest level of BP at baseline had the lowest cognitive scores. A similar approach, with an even longer duration of follow-up of 25 years, was within the framework of the Honolulu–Asia Aging Study (HAAS).[10] Among over 3700 men followed since 1965, the relative risk (RR) for dementia was 3.8 (95% confidence interval (CI) 1.6–8.7) for those with a diastolic BP of 90–94 mmHg at baseline, and 4.3 (95% CI 1.7–10.8) for those with a diastolic BP of ≥95 mmHg compared with those with a diastolic BP of 80–89 mmHg at baseline. Compared with those with a systolic BP of 110–139 mmHg at baseline, the risk for dementia was 4.8 (95% CI 2.0–11.0) in those with systolic BP ≥160 mmHg at baseline. This relationship was most apparent in those patients who were never treated with BP-lowering drugs. A similar relationship was found in both a Swedish and French study, both with about 20 years of follow-up.[11,12]

Thus, the evidence from several large population-based prospective studies with a long-term follow-up of more than 15 years suggests that BP levels measured in mid life (usually 10–25 years before the onset of dementia) are related to significantly increased risk for AD. Although spurious associations are plausible in these cross-sectional studies on BP and cognition and dementia, these prospective longitudinal studies seem to be unequivocal.

BP-lowering drugs and AD: prospective population-based studies

In the large study (although not a randomized clinical trial) of the Kungsholmen Project, about 1300 non-demented persons at baseline were followed for an average period of 3 years.[13] It was shown that in the subpopulation treated for hypertension with diuretics, incidence of AD was significantly reduced compared with hypertensives who had no treatment (RR = 0.6, 95% CI 0.3–1.2). In the Rotterdam Study, in which over 7000 individuals were followed to record incidence of dementia, treatment of BP (irrespective of the type) was related to a non-significant reduction in the incidence of AD (RR = 0.9, 95% CI 0.6–1.4).[14]

The limitations of these studies were that information on drug use was not available throughout the entire study period, the duration of treatment was unknown, and, more importantly, confounding-by-indication may have played an important role: e.g. due to the possibility that users of BP-lowering agents were in better health compared with non-users (and as such this may have led to a reduced incidence of AD among users). The overall results, however, seem to be encouraging in suggesting that some treatment of hypertension impedes progression of cognitive decline. Needless to say, these findings should be confirmed in properly designed double-blind randomized clinical trials.

BP-lowering drugs and AD: double-blind randomized clinical trials

To date, at least four major randomized, placebo-controlled hypertension trials have included substudies focusing on the course of cognition during treatment and incidence of dementia. The first trial was the Systolic Hypertension in the Elderly Program (SHEP),[15] in which about 2000 patients aged ≥60 years old with isolated hypertension (systolic BP ≥160 mmHg and diastolic BP <90 mmHg) were enrolled for placebo or active chlorthalidone treatment. All participants underwent extensive neuropsychologic testing. The outcome was disappointing; neither the evolution of cognitive function nor the incidence of dementia was significantly different between the active and placebo groups. In contrast, in the Syst-Eur placebo controlled randomized trial,[16] in patients with isolated systolic hypertension treated with the calcium antagonist nitrendipine, a reduction of 7 mmHg in systolic and 3.2 mmHg in diastolic BP over 3.9 years significantly reduced the incidence of AD by 50%. The absolute risk reduction was 3 cases per 100 patient-years. A 2-year open-label extension of the trial showed similar results, with a 55% reduction in dementia incidence for those receiving long-term therapy ($p < 0.001$).[17] This is the only trial in which a significant decrease in the incidence of AD was apparent.

The PROGRESS study was a randomized, double-blind trial among 6105 people with a prior history of cerebrovascular events.[18] Participants were assigned to active treatment, which comprised perindopril for all participants and indapamide for those with neither an indication for nor a contraindication to a diuretic or matching placebo(s). Results from that study demonstrated a reduction, over 3.9 years of follow-up, in risk of dementia from 7.1 to 6.3% (non-significant) and in cognitive decline from 11 to 9.1%. It is possible that the benefit was due to the prevention of recurrent stroke.

In the SCOPE study, candesartan-based antihypertensive treatment (an angiotensin receptor II antagonist) in elderly patients with mild to moderately elevated BP conferred a reduction in cardiovascular events, cognitive decline, and dementia.[19] This was a prospective, double-blind, randomized trial of almost 5000 patients aged 70–89 years old, with systolic BP 160–179 mmHg, and/or diastolic BP 90–99 mmHg, and a Mini-Mental State Examination (MMSE) test score ≥24. However, this study had a special design, such that, in patients who needed BP-lowering drugs, these could be added, despite not being assigned to the active treatment group. As a consequence, active antihypertensive therapy was also extensively used in the control group (84%) and the BP difference between cases and controls was only 3.2/1.6 mmHg, and there was no demonstrable effect on cognition over a mean of 3.7 years. Because of this atypical design, both the active and placebo groups exhibited decreases in BP of about 20/10 mmHg: thus, both groups were, in effect, treatment groups.

What can be recommended to the patients?

No single trial provides exact answers to the questions of whether or not to treat an AD patient with BP-lowering agents (with respect to cognition) and to which level BP should be lowered. Available information points towards a preventive effect for AD of BP-lowering drugs. However, this concerns only patients without dementia, and may not apply to the patients with dementia we see daily. Another complicating factor is that all studies that have investigated cognition with respect to BP-lowering treatment comprised patients with symptomatic (cardio)vascular diseases. In other words, do we recognize patients with AD in these studies? For the moment, this seems not to be the case. Extrapolating findings from the earlier-mentioned studies suggests that treating BP may prevent progression of cognitive decline in patients with AD. It may be wise to use this type of treatment only for those who are at the beginning of the disease and are able to live relatively independently. Obviously, caution should be taken in those patients who are already at a more severe stage of the disease. It is reasonable to assume that use of BP-lowering agents in patients that already experience a decrease in BP during the end stage of the disease will harm the brain by inducing further hypoperfusion.

CHOLESTEROL

High cholesterol is an established risk factor for cardiovascular disease; much less is clear with respect to cerebrovascular disease. However, there are some indications from prospective studies that a history of high cholesterol may play a role in the etiology of AD. In the aforementioned HAAS, cholesterol levels were measured in late life and mid life (approximately 20 years before late life).[20] After adjusting for possible confounding factors, a strong linear association was found for increasing late-life HDL (high-density lipoprotein) cholesterol levels and an increasing number of neocortical neuritic plaques, analyzed at autopsy (5th vs 1st quintile: count ratio = 2.30, 95% CI 1.05–5.06). Trends were similar for the mid-life HDL cholesterol levels. Additional circumstantial evidence comes from a large pharmacoepidemiologic case-control study that found a reduced risk in the incidence of dementia in not-otherwise-specified statin users.[21] Other researchers have failed to replicate these findings.[22] These findings suggest the role for cholesterol in the etiology of AD is equivocal, but the definitive answer must come from prospective trials.

Cholesterol-lowering drugs and AD: trial

The most convincing proof for a role of cholesterol in the etiology of AD would be a reduction of the incidence of dementia in the active treated group of a double-blind clinical trial. In the PROSPER study, about 6000 individuals aged 70–82 years old were followed for a mean period of 3.2 years; half of them were randomized to receive pravastatin.[23] Cognitive function declined at the same rate in both treatment groups. For example, there were no significant differences between the two groups in the difference between the last on-treatment and the second baseline value for the MMSE score (difference = 0.06, 95% CI –0.04 to 0.16, $p = 0.26$). It remains uncertain why cholesterol lowering appears successful in the primary and secondary prevention of vascular events and why cognitive status remains largely unaffected. One possibility could be due to the trial design. Several cognitive rating scales were used here but a complete dementia work-up was not carried out. Recently, a small randomized, placebo-controlled, double-blind trial provided evidence on the effects of the daily administration of 80 mg simvastatin in 44 normocholesterolemic patients with AD. The authors found that decreases in MMSE scores were significantly retarded over time in the treated group compared with the control group.[24] Thus, it was suggested for the first time that treatment with a statin reduces the deterioration of cognitive function; however, the underlying mechanisms remain to be elucidated.

What can be recommended to the patients?

There is no clear evidence of any beneficial effect on cognition of cholesterol-lowering drugs such as the statins. This was also the conclusion of the Cochrane collaborators in a large meta-analysis of available data on this topic.[25] While further studies are being pursued, statins should currently be given only for the prevention of new vascular events. Results from studies in the elderly suggest that there is no lower threshold for cholesterol levels to be treated with the purpose of reducing vascular risk.

DIABETES MELLITUS

Diabetes is a major risk factor for stroke, which is only partially mediated through hypertension. There is conflicting evidence concerning the effect of diabetes on cognitive function. In the Third National Health and Nutrition Examination Survey (NHANES III), there was no apparent association between diabetes and cognitive function. However these patients were between 30 and 60 years of age;[26] in the elderly, diabetes has been associated with cognitive impairment. In two large epidemiologic studies – one involving the Mayo Clinic cohort and the other the Rotterdam Study – diabetes was associated with an increased risk for incident AD.[27,28] In an analysis of over 6000 elderly persons, there was a positive association between diabetes and dementia (odds ratio (OR) = 1.3, 95% CI 1.0–1.9). Furthermore, strong associations were found between dementia and diabetes treated with insulin (OR = 3.2, 95% CI 1.4–7.5).

Glucose-lowering drugs and AD: trial

As for the other vascular risk factors, the definitive answer for the involvement of diabetes in the pathophysiology of AD should come from prospective trials. To date, no such trials, which also include extensive neuropsychologic testing, have been done, but there is one that has just recently been launched, known as the ADVANCE study.[29] In this trial, BP lowering was combined with intensive glucose lowering. Glucose lowering in these patients was also shown to reduce microvascular disease. The secondary outcomes include dementia.

What can be recommended to the patients?

Although diabetes is an obvious risk factor for vascular disease and AD, surprisingly little is known on the treatment of diabetes with respect to the development of AD. It appears trials on this topic have not previously been executed. Strict glucose control targeting a glycated hemoglobin A_{1c} concentration of 7.0% seems fair for a patient at the early stages of AD, mainly for the prevention of diabetic complications.

HOMOCYSTEINE

Perhaps, unsurprisingly, the link between homocysteine and cognition is tenuous at best. A few studies have reported an inverse association between plasma total homocysteine concentrations and simultaneously assessed cognitive function,[30–32] whereas another study showed that plasma homocysteine was not related to cognitive decline.[33] In addition, it is unclear whether actual homocysteine levels reflect lifetime homocysteine exposure, since plasma homocysteine levels in subjects with cognitive impairment or dementia may be elevated due to poor nutrition and vitamin deficiencies. To overcome this problem, the relationship between plasma total homocysteine level and incident dementia was investigated in the Framingham Study.[34] The results showed that increase in 1 SD homocysteine value (at baseline) was associated with an RR for the development of AD of 1.4 (95% CI 1.1–1.9). Hyperhomocysteinemia (plasma homocysteine, >14 µmol/L) was associated with an almost doubled risk for AD (RR = 1.9, 95% CI 1.2–3.0). The risk of AD attributable to a plasma homocysteine level in the highest age-specific quartile was estimated at 16%.

Homocysteine-lowering drugs and AD: trial

Fortunately, homocysteine can be lowered rather easily by supplementing diets with folic acid. A common practice in the United States since 1998 is the supplementation with folic acid of grain products. Indeed, previous studies in persons not diagnosed with AD suggest that high-dose vitamin supplementation can reduce plasma levels of homocysteine by 25%, but this does not correspond to an attendant increase in cognition. In preparation for a large multi-center trial to determine whether homocysteine reduction slows progression in persons with AD, a feasibility study was conducted to determine the impact of high-dose vitamin supplementation on fasting and post-methionine-loading homocysteine in US subjects with AD.[35] This was done in the presence of folic acid fortification of grain products. The question was also asked whether high-dose supplements reduced homocysteine levels in users of daily multivitamins. Among 69 subjects, the high-dose vitamin regimen was associated with a significant reduction in fasting and post-methionine-loading homocysteine. Reductions were greater in the subgroup not using multivitamins, but were also significant in the multivitamin users. Unfortunately, measures of cognitive status were not incorporated in this study.

To date, there is only one preliminary report on the effect of folic acid supplementation on cognition among dementia patients.[36] A small placebo-controlled trial on the effects of folic acid 10 mg/day vs placebo in 11 patients (although only 7 completed the study) with dementia and low-normal folic acid levels was conducted. The magnitude of change between baseline and second testing was not statistically significant between the two groups, although the treated group did worse. Larger studies are necessary before empirically administering folic acid to patients already suffering from dementia.

What can be recommended to the patients?

Again, firm recommendations cannot be made for folic acid supplementation (with or without vitamin B_6 or B_{12}) in treating cognitive decline in patients with existing mild-to-moderate AD. Despite the promising results from the prospective studies, results from the single small trial are disappointing. Notwithstanding methodologic flaws in these studies, it is plausible that intervention in an already ongoing disease is something completely different than performing follow-up studies in which the relationship between the plasma level of a certain risk factor and an outcome is investigated.

SUMMARY

1. High BP and cholesterol levels should be treated in those mild-to-moderately affected AD patients in whom the treating physician finds it useful to prevent cardiovascular events. The levels at which treatment should be started are not defined in this setting, but it seems reasonable to keep in line with general recommendations in order to prevent cardiovascular symptoms (systolic BP $\geq$140 mmHg and/or diastolic BP $\geq$90 mmHg; total cholesterol $\geq$5.0 mmol/L (or LDL (low-density lipoprotein)-cholesterol $\geq$3.2 mmol/L)). Presumably, cognitive decline is inhibited by BP-lowering agents and statins, in mild-to-moderately affected AD, but there is only limited evidence. To date, too little is known as to which class of

BP-lowering drugs should be used and to which level BP can be safely reduced in elderly demented patients. Treating hypertension seems more important than the choice of agent. For cholesterol, there are currently no such indications.

2. Diabetes should be treated, targeting a glycated hemoglobin A_{1c} concentration of 7.0–8% in patients with AD in order to prevent disabling diabetic complications. There is no evidence of any beneficial effect on cognition of strict glucose control in patients with AD.

3. Treatment of homocysteine with 5–10 mg folic acid (with or without vitamins B_6 and B_{12}) can effectively reduce homocysteine levels in AD patients. To date, the effects on cognition are under scrutiny. One should never begin treating without knowledge of the patient's vitamin B_{12} levels.

REFERENCES

1. Skoog I, Kalaria RN, Breteler MMB. Vascular factors and Alzheimer's disease. Alzheimer Dis Assoc Disord 1999;13:S106–114.

2. De Leeuw F-E, de Groot JC, Oudkerk M, et al. A follow-up study of blood pressure and cerebral white matter lesions. Ann Neurol 1999;46:827–833.

3. De Leeuw F-E, de Groot JC, Oudkerk M, et al. Hypertension and cerebral white matter lesions in a prospective cohort study. Brain 2002;125:765–772.

4. Vermeer SE, Prins ND, den Heijer T, et al. Silent brain infarcts and the risk of dementia and cognitive decline. N Engl J Med 2003;348:1215–1222.

5. Seux ML, Forette F. Effects of hypertension and its treatment on mental function. Curr Hypertens Rep 1999;1:232–237

.6. Skoog I, Lernfelt B, Landahl S, et al. 15-year longitudinal study of blood pressure and dementia. Lancet 1996;347:1141–1145.

7. Qiu C, von Strauss E, Winblad B, Fratiglioni L. Decline in blood pressure over time and risk of dementia: a longitudinal study from the Kungsholmen project. Stroke 2004; 35(8):1810–1815. Epub 2004 Jul 01.

8. Petitti DB, Crooks VC, Buckwalter JG, Chiu V. Blood pressure levels before dementia. Arch Neurol 2005;62: 112–116.

9. Elias ME, Wolf PA, D'Agostino RB, Cobb J, White LR. Untreated blood pressure level is inversely related to cognitive functioning: the Framingham study. Am J Epidemiol 1993; 138:353–364.

10. Launer LJ, Ross GW, Petrovitch H, et al. Midlife blood pressure and dementia: the Honolulu–Asia aging study. Neurobiol Aging 2000;21:49–55.

11. Kilander L, Nyman H, Boberg M, Hansson L, Lithell H. Hypertension is related to cognitive impairment: a 20-year follow-up of 999 men. Hypertension 1998;31:780–786.

12. Tzourio C, Dufouil C, Ducimetière P, Alperovitch A. Cognitive decline in individuals with high blood pressure. Neurolog 1999;53:1948–1952.

13. Guo Z, Fratiglioni L, Winblad B, Viitanen M. Blood pressure and performance on the Mini-Mental State Examination in the very old: cross-sectional and longitudinal data from the Kungsholmen Project. Am J Epidemiol 1997;145:1106–1113.

14. Ruitenberg A, Skoog I, Ott A, et al. Blood pressure and risk of dementia: results from the Rotterdam study and the Gothenburg H-70 Study. Dement Geriatr Cogn Disord 2001;12:33–39.

15. Applegiate WB, Pressels S, Wittes J, et al. Impact of the treatment of isolated systolic hypertension on behavioral variables: results from the Systolic Hypertension in the Elderly Program. Arch Intern Med 1994; 154:2154–2160.

16. Forette F, Seux M-L, Staessen JA, et al. Prevention of dementia in randomised double-blind placebo-controlled Systolic Hypertension in Europe (Syst-Eur) trial. Lancet 1998; 352:1347–1351.

17. Forette F, Seux ML, Staessen JA, et al. Systolic Hypertension in Europe Investigators. The prevention of dementia with antihypertensive treatment: new evidence from the Systolic Hypertension in Europe (Syst-Eur) study. Arch Intern Med 2002;162: 2046–2052.

18. Tzourio C, Anderson C, Chapman N, et al, for the PROGRESS Collaborative Group. Effects of blood pressure lowering with perindopril and indapamide therapy on dementia and cognitive decline in patients with cerebrovascular disease. Arch Intern Med 2003;163:1069–1075.

19. Lithell H, Hansson L, Skoog I, et al. The Study on Cognition and Prognosis in the Elderly (SCOPE): principal results of a randomized double-blind intervention trial. J Hypertens 2003;21:875–886.

20. Launer LJ, White LR, Petrovitch H, Ross GW, Curb JD. Cholesterol and neuropathologic markers of AD: a population-based autopsy study. Neurology 2001;57:1447–1452.

21. Jick H, Zornberg GL, Jick SS, Seshadri S, Drachman DA. Statins and the risk of dementia. Lancet 2000;356:1627–1631.

22. Li G, Higdon R, Kukull WA, et al. Statin therapy and risk of dementia in the elderly: a community-based prospective cohort study. Neurology 2004;63:1624–1628.

23. Shepherd J, Blauw GJ, Murphy MB, et al; PROSPER study group. PROspective Study of Pravastatin in the Elderly at Risk. Pravastatin in elderly individuals at risk of vascular disease (PROSPER): a randomised controlled trial. Lancet 2002;360: 1623–1630.

24. Simons M, Schwarzler F, Lutjohann D, et al. Treatment with simvastatin in normocholesterolemic patients with Alzheimer's disease: a 26-week randomized, placebo-controlled, double-blind trial. Ann Neurol 2002;52:346–350.

25. Scott HD, Laake K. Statins for the prevention of Alzheimer's disease. Cochrane Database Syst Rev 2001; (4):CD003160.

26. Pavlik VN, Hyman DJ, Doody R. Cardiovascular risk factors and cognitive function in adults 30–59 years of age (NHANES III). Neuroepidemiology 2005;24(1–2):42–50. Epub 2005.

27. Leibson CL, Rocca WA, Hanson VA, et al. Risk of dementia among persons with diabetes mellitus: a population-based cohort study. Am J Epidemiol 1997;145:301–308.

28. Ott A, Stolk RP, van Harskamp F, et al. Diabetes mellitus and the risk of dementia: The Rotterdam Study. Neurology 1999;53:1937–1942.

29. ADVANCE Collaborative Group (Chalmers J, Ferrannini E, Glasziou P et al). Rationale and design of the ADVANCE study: a randomised trial of blood pressure lowering and intensive glucose control in high-risk individuals with type 2 diabetes mellitus. Action in Diabetes and Vascular Disease: PreterAx and DiamicroN Modified-Release Controlled Evaluation.

30. Riggs KM, Spiro A III, Tucker K, Rush D. Relations of vitamin B-12, vitamin B-6, folate, and homocysteine to cognitive performance in the Normative Aging Study. Am J Clin Nutr 1996;63:306–314.

31. Bell IR, Edman JS, Selhub J, et al. Plasma homocysteine in vascular disease and in nonvascular dementia of depressed elderly people. Acta Psychiatr Scand 1992;86:386–390.

32 Clarke R, Smith AD, Jobst KA, et al. Folate, vitamin B12, and serum total homocysteine levels in confirmed Alzheimer disease. Arch Neurol 1998;55(11):1449–1455.

33. Ravaglia G, Forti P, Maioli F, et al. Blood homocysteine and vitamin B levels are not associated with cognitive skills in healthy normally ageing subjects. J Nutr Health Aging 2000;4:218–222.

34 Seshadri S, Beiser A, Selhub J, et al. Plasma homocysteine as a risk factor for dementia and Alzheimer's disease. N Engl J Med 2002;346:476–483.

35 Aisen PS, Egelko S, Andrews H, et al. A pilot study of vitamins to lower plasma homocysteine levels in Alzheimer disease. Am J Geriatr Psychiatry 2003;11:246–249.

36 Sommer BR, Hoff AL, Costa M. Folic acid supplementation in dementia: a preliminary report. J Geriatr Psychiatry Neurol 2003;16:156–159.

10
Cognitive dysfunction in multiple sclerosis

Julie A Bobholz and Angela Gleason

Our understanding of cognitive dysfunction in multiple sclerosis (MS) has advanced significantly during the past few decades. Studies have suggested that nearly half of all patients with this disease will experience cognitive decline, making cognitive dysfunction one of the most common symptoms of MS. This chapter will provide an overview of recent developments in understanding:

1. the characteristics of cognitive dysfunction, including pattern and course
2. the impact cognitive dysfunction has on daily living
3. neurobehavioral and neuroimaging correlates of cognitive deficits
4. recently examined treatment options.

CHARACTERISTICS OF COGNITIVE DYSFUNCTION IN MULTIPLE SCLEROSIS

Estimates of the prevalence of cognitive dysfunction in MS vary significantly across studies,[1–3] although well-designed neuropsychologic studies in MS have shown prevalence rates as high as 65%.[1] Although the development of MS-related cognitive decline can occur anytime throughout the course of MS, some researchers have found signs of decline relatively early in the disease. In a recent investigation of patients diagnosed with probable MS ($n = 67$), 54% of the sample showed evidence for discrete cognitive impairment on one or two neuropsychologic tests, with impairment defined as performance one standard deviation (1 SD) below the normative mean.[4] Lyon-Caen and colleagues[5] suggested that as many as 85% of patients with clinically definite multiple sclerosis of less than 2 years' duration have some degree of cognitive impairment.

Pattern of cognitive deficits

Significant heterogeneity in cognitive dysfunction can be seen across patients with MS, yet cross-sectional and longitudinal studies have consistently identified deficits in areas of recent memory, working memory, information-processing speed, executive functions, verbal abstraction, and visuospatial perception.[1,3,6–8] This chapter reviews most recent developments in this area of MS research.

Memory decline is one of the most frequently reported cognitive changes in MS, affecting approximately 40–60% of individuals with MS.[9] In general, explicit memory tends to be most affected with relatively spared semantic memory, autobiographical memory (for personal semantic information), and implicit memory. There has been debate in the literature regarding the extent to which deficits in encoding or retrieval operations account for the memory disturbance. In studies controlling for initial learning by requiring all subjects to reach a certain criterion for performance on learning trials, patients with MS generally show similar levels of delayed recall, although they require more learning trials to initially reach criterion.[10–12] In a recent study, Thornton and colleagues[13] used an encoding specificity paradigm to systematically study the encoding and retrieval aspects of memory in MS. Results suggested that MS patients were able to recall words that had associations within a pre-existing semantic network (e.g. target word *queen* presented with retrieval cue *king*), but were less able to recall words that required new associations during encoding (target word *cold* presented with retrieval cue *ground*). The authors suggest that memory deficits in MS may be related to deficits in binding of contextual information during the encoding phase of learning. The deficit in initial acquisition has also been proposed to be related to information-processing deficits, as well as difficulties with efficiently encoding information,[14,15] rather than repetition of information per se.[16] Arnett[17] found that fewer patients with MS scored in the impaired range on a measure of story memory when the stories were presented at a slower rate.

In addition to impaired explicit memory, deficits in recall of autobiographical episodic information have also been demonstrated, with an estimated 60% of patients with advanced MS (average time since diagnosis of 21.4 years) showing a temporal gradient of greater memory impairment for recent events.[18]

Impaired attention and processing speed has been reported in several studies examining cognitive dysfunction in MS.[1,19–22] In addition, studies have demonstrated deficits on measures of executive functions, including abstract reasoning and concept formation skills.[23–25]

In a well-designed, long-term, and controlled natural history study, Amato and colleagues[8] compared 45 MS and 65 matched control subjects on a battery of neuropsychologic measures over a 10-year interval. At the baseline examination, the MS sample showed deficits on tasks of verbal memory, abstract reasoning, and linguistic processes. At the end of the 10-year interval, additional deficits were seen on tasks of attention and short-term spatial memory. The prevalence of cognitive dysfunction increased from 26 to 56% over the 10-year retest interval.

IMPACT OF COGNITIVE DYSFUNCTION ON DAILY LIVING

Research has suggested that cognitive dysfunction can have a devastating impact on patients' ability to maintain employment, independent living skills, and social relationships. In the Amato longitudinal study described above, 17 of the 25 MS patients who were mild or moderately impaired on cognitive examination had to modify or discontinue their work activity. Furthermore, 18 of the cognitively impaired subjects showed severe limits in social interactions and required assistance in their personal lives. In contrast, only 2 members of the cognitively intact group showed similar limitations.[8]

Employment

Unemployment is high in MS, with some estimates as high as 70–80% of patients are unemployed 5 years following initial diagnosis.[26,27] Considering an estimated 60% of people are employed when diagnosed with MS, only 20–30% are working 10–15 years later. Yet, other studies have found that nearly half of the unemployed people with MS wish to return to work. The self-reported reasons for unemployment include factors such as impact of fatigue, stress in the workplace, and cognitive changes.[28] In fact, individuals with cognitive impairment are more likely to have problems with employment compared to those without cognitive dysfunction.[29,30] With this data in mind, accommodations in the workplace and adjustments in responsibilities will increase the chance that MS patients continue working, and some employers are already making these adjustments.[31]

Driving

Several recent investigations have raised concern about driving safety in patients with MS. Shawaryn and colleagues[32] found that performance on a speeded, complex measure of working memory (Paced Auditory Serial Addition Test; PASAT) was significantly correlated with overall performances on a variety of computerized instruments designed to assess driving skill. Similarly, another investigation found that accident rates on a driving simulator test were significantly correlated with PASAT performance but not with physical functioning in a sample of 31 patients with relapsing-remitting MS.[33] A recent review of archival records from the Department of Motor Vehicles over the past 5 consecutive years found that patients with MS who demonstrated cognitive impairment on neuropsychologic measures had a higher incidence of motor vehicle accidents (54%) when compared with MS patients without cognitive impairment (7%) and control subjects (6%).[34] Although this study involved a relatively small sample of patients (13 MS patients with cognitive impairment, 14 MS patients without cognitive impairment, and 17 healthy controls), it highlights the potential increased safety risk in cognitively impaired drivers with MS.

Quality of life

Efforts to quantify the impact MS has on daily living and quality of life have included the development of inventories such as the Health-Related Quality of Life, Multiple Sclerosis Quality of Life, Functional Assessment of Multiple Sclerosis, and the MS Quality of Life-54. Studies have shown that decreased quality of life is associated with increased disease burden on the MS Functional Composite,[35] magnetic resonance (MR) brain lesions and atrophy,[36] and on measures of cognitive and emotional functions.[37,38]

CORRELATES WITH COGNITIVE DYSFUNCTION IN MULTIPLE SCLEROSIS

Disease variables and gender

Disease variables such as disease duration and level of physical disability have been inconsistently associated with cognitive dysfunction in MS.[39–42] Most studies showing lack of correlation with disease variables have used cross-sectional research designs. In contrast, Amato and colleagues found that, after a 10-year study interval, extent of cognitive impairment was associated with degree of physical disability, progressive disease course, and increased age.[8]

Researchers have recognized that patients with secondary progressive disease show greater cognitive impairment on average than patients with relapsing-remitting MS.[43,44] A recent retrospective cross-sectional study of 391 patients with clinically definite MS revealed greater relative risk for cognitive impairment for patients with secondary progressive disease compared with patients with relapsing-remitting disease across multiple cognitive domains.[45] These differences were demonstrated across all six cognitive factors from the Wechsler Adult Intelligence Scale – Third Edition (WAIS-III) and Wechsler Memory Scale – Third Edition (WMS-III): verbal comprehension, perceptual organization, processing speed, working memory, auditory memory, and visual memory. Patients with primary progressive MS have also been shown to perform poorer on measures of verbal learning compared with patients with relapsing-remitting MS.[46] The impact course has on cognitive dysfunction is relatively consistent with investigations that have shown the greatest degree of MR pathology in patients with primary and secondary progressive course.[47,48]

Although MS more commonly affects women, MS-related cognitive dysfunction appears more prominent in men.[49] In a series of MS studies, Beatty and colleagues[30,49,50] reported that men performed more poorly than women on neuropsychologic measures of verbal memory, nonverbal memory, processing speed, verbal fluency, facial recognition, visual construction, and novel problem solving. These differences were not associated with age at diagnosis or

Glatiramer acetate had no significant effect on cognitive functions in a multicenter, randomized, placebo-controlled study following 1- and 2-year intervals.[89]

Symptomatic agents

A few studies have examined the impact of cholinesterase inhibitor therapy on cognitive functions and have found positive treatment effects.[90,91] Recently, Krupp and colleagues[92] reported improved memory in MS patients treated with donepezil, as part of a randomized, double-blind, placebo-controlled clinical trial. Patients ($n = 69$) were assigned to either a treatment or placebo group, then tested cognitively at baseline and after 24 weeks. Whereas memory performance improved in the treatment group, other cognitive measures did not improve with treatment.

A few studies have also shown positive effects from amantadine. Cohen and Fischer[93] found improved performance on the Stroop task when treated with amantadine, whereas Geisler et al[94] showed improved written speed on the Symbol Digit Modalities Test with amantadine.

Patzold and colleagues[95] assessed changes in physical disability (Expanded Disability Status Scale; EDSS) and the MSFC (Multiple Sclerosis Functional Composite) in a sample of MS patients receiving methylprednisolone over a 20-day interval. The results of this controlled study suggested that all three components of the MSFC – including the PASAT (Paced Auditory Serial Addition Test) – were sensitive to changes in clinical activity, with significant improvement noted following treatment. In contrast, the EDSS did not change significantly.

In a double-blind pilot study assessing the effect of Prokarin on fatigue, the Prokarin-treated group experienced significant improvements after 12 weeks on the MSFC, including the PASAT.[96] Results from this study are encouraging, although the sample sizes were small. In contrast, results of a randomized, double-blind, placebo-controlled, crossover trial of oral 4-aminopyridine with 54 progressive MS patients failed to show significant improvement in cognitive functions.[97]

Rehabilitation techniques

Cognitive rehabilitation techniques are designed to either restore functions or develop strategies to compensate for cognitive dysfunction. There have been some promising results to suggest that cognitive rehabilitation in MS is effective. Strategies aimed at adaptation and coping with cognitive dysfunction may be helpful. For example, cognitive reframing of a problem enhances use of compensation strategies. Patients can also have improved functions with the use of organization, planning, and memory aids.[98–100]

Jonsson et al.[101] compared cognitive performances by MS patients who were randomly assigned to a treatment group (direct training program with compensatory strategies and therapy) with those assigned to a non-treatment group. After 6 months, the group who received intervention performed significantly better on a measure of visuospatial memory. Other researchers have reported positive effects of computer-based retraining programs.[102,103]

Finally, cognitive-behavioral therapy has been shown to be effective in improving cognitive functions.[104,105] Typically, this form of therapy included enhancement of insight with education, social skills training, behavioral modification techniques, and relaxation strategies.

SUMMARY

This chapter highlights some of the most recent literature pertaining to cognitive dysfunction in MS. With the past few decades of research in this area, there is general consensus that cognitive dysfunction does occur in MS and that the prevalence is fairly high. Given the impact cognitive dysfunction has on daily living skills, efforts continue to identify correlates with cognitive dysfunction and treatment options. Future research will build on this strong foundation of knowledge, with the ultimate hope that healthcare providers will have effective treatment options to offer these individuals.

REFERENCES

1. Rao SM, Leo GJ, Bernardin L, Unverzagt F. Cognitive dysfunction in multiple sclerosis. I. Frequency, patterns, and prediction. Neurology 1991;41(5):685–691.

2. Peyser JM, Edwards KR, Poser CM, Filskov SB. Cognitive function in patients with multiple sclerosis. Arch Neurol 1980;37(9):577–579.

3. Piras MR, Magnano I, Canu ED, et al. Longitudinal study of cognitive dysfunction in multiple sclerosis: neuropsychological, neuroradiological, and neurophysiological findings. J Neurol Neurosurg Psychiatry 2003; 74(7):878–885.

4. Achiron A, Barak Y. Cognitive impairment in probable multiple sclerosis. J Neurol Neurosurg Psychiatry 2003;74(4):443–446.

5. Lyon-Caen O, Jouvent R, Hauser S, et al. Cognitive function in recent-onset demyelinating diseases. Arch Neurol 1986;43(11):1138–1141.

6. Ryan L, Clark C, Klonoff H. Patterns of cognitive impairment in relapsing-remitting multiple sclerosis and their relationship to neuropathology on magnetic resonance images. Neuropsychology 1996;10: 176–193.

7. Amato MP, Ponziani G, Pracucci G, et al. Cognitive impairment in early-onset multiple sclerosis. Pattern, predictors, and impact on everyday life in a 4-year follow-up. Arch Neurol 1995;52(2):168–172.

8. Amato MP, Ponziani G, Siracusa G, Sorbi S. Cognitive dysfunction in early-onset multiple sclerosis: a reappraisal after 10 years. Arch Neurol 2001;58(10):1602–1606.

9 Rao SM, Grafman J, Dijkerman HC. Memory dysfunction in multiple sclerosis: its relation to working memory, semantic encoding, and implicit learning. Neuropsychology 1993;7:364–374.

10. DeLuca J, Barbieri-Berger S, Johnson SK. The nature of memory impairments in multiple sclerosis: acquisition versus retrieval. J Clin Exp Neuropsychol 1994;16(2):183–189.

11. DeLuca J, Gaudino EA, Diamond BJ, Christodoulou C, Engel RA. Acquisition and storage deficits in multiple sclerosis. J Clin Exp Neuropsychol 1998;20(3):376–390.

12. Demaree HA, Gaudino EA, DeLuca J, Ricker JH. Learning impairment is associated with recall ability in multiple sclerosis. J Clin Exp Neuropsychol 2000;22(6):865–873.

13. Thornton AE, Raz N, Tucke KA. Memory in multiple sclerosis: contextual encoding deficits. J Int Neuropsychol Soc 2002;8(3):395–409.

14. Archibald CJ, Fisk JD. Information processing efficiency in patients with multiple sclerosis. J Clin Exp Neuropsychol 2000;22(5):686–701.

15. DeLuca J, Chelune GJ, Tulsky DS, Lengenfelder J, Chiaravalloti ND. Is speed of processing or working memory the primary information processing deficit in multiple sclerosis? J Clin Exp Neurophyschol 2004;26:550–562.

16. Chiaravalloti ND, Demaree H, Gaudino EA, DeLuca J. Can the repetition effect maximize learning in multiple sclerosis? Clin Rehabil 2003;17(1):58–68.

17. Arnett PA. Speed of presentation influences story recall in college students and persons with multiple sclerosis. Arch Clin Neuropsychol 2004;19:507–523.

18. Kenealy PM, Beaumont JG, Lintern TC, Murrell RC. Autobiographical memory in advanced multiple sclerosis: assessment of episodic and personal semantic memory across three time spans. J Int Neuropsychol Soc 2002;8(6):855–860.

19. Kujala P, Portin R, Revonsuo A, Ruutiainen J. Attention related performance in two cognitively different subgroups of patients with multiple sclerosis. J Neurol Neurosurg Psychiatry 1995;59(1):77–82.

20. DeLuca J, Johnson SK, Natelson BH. Information processing efficiency in chronic fatigue syndrome and multiple sclerosis. Arch Neurol 1993;50(3):301–304.

21. Demaree HA, DeLuca J, Gaudino EA, Diamond BJ. Speed of information processing as a key deficit in multiple sclerosis: implications for rehabilitation. J Neurol Neurosurg Psychiatry 1999;67(5):661–663.

22. Litvan I, Grafman J, Vendrell P, Martinez JM. Slowed information processing in multiple sclerosis. Arch Neurol 1988;45(3):281–285.

23. Foong J, Rozewicz L, Quaghebeur G, et al. Executive function in multiple sclerosis. The role of frontal lobe pathology. Brain 1997;120(Pt 1):15–26.

24. Mendozzi L, Pugnetti L, Saccani M, Motta A. Frontal lobe dysfunction in multiple sclerosis as assessed by means of Lurian tasks: effect of age at onset. J Neurol Sci 1993;115(Suppl):S42–S50.

25. Beatty WW, Monson N. Problem solving by patients with multiple sclerosis: comparison of performance on the Wisconsin and California Card Sorting Tests. J Int Neuropsychol Soc 1996;2(2):134–140.

26. Kornblith AM, LeRocca NG, Baum K. Employment in individuals with multiple sclerosis. Int J Rehabil Res 1986;9:155–165.

27. LaRocca NG, Kalb R, Gregg K. A program to facilitate retention of employment among persons with multiple sclerosis. Work: A Journal of Prevention, Assessment and Rehabilitation 1996;7:37–46.

28. Johnson KL, Yorkston KM, Klasner ER, et al. The cost and benefits of employment: a qualitative study of experiences of persons with multiple sclerosis. Arch Phys Med Rehabil 2004;85(2):201–209.

29. Rao SM, Leo GJ, Ellington L, et al. Cognitive dysfunction in multiple sclerosis. II. Impact on employment and social functioning. Neurology 1991;41(5):692–696.

30. Beatty WW, Blanco C, Wilbanks S, Paul R. Demographic, clinical and cognitive characteristics of multiple sclerosis patients who continue to work. J Neurol Rehab 1995; 9:167–173.

31. Johnson KL, Yorkston KM, Klasner ER, et al. The cost and benefits of employment: a qualitative study of experiences of persons with multiple sclerosis. Arch Phys Med Rehabil 2004;85(2):201–209.

32. Shawaryn M, Schultheis M, Garay E, DeLuca J. Assessing functional status: Exploring the relationship between the Multiple Sclerosis Functional Composite and driving. Arch Phys Med Rehabil 2002;83: 1123–1129.

33. Kotterba S, Orth M, Eren E, Fangerau T, Sindern E. Assessment of driving performance in patients with relapsing-remitting multiple sclerosis by a driving simulator. Eur Neurol 2003;50(3):160–164.

34. Schultheis MT, Garay E, Millis SR, DeLuca J. Motor vehicle crashes and violations among drivers with multiple sclerosis. Arch Phys Med Rehabil 2002;83(8):1175–1178.

35. Miller DM, Rudick RA, Cutter G, Baier M, Fischer JS. Clinical significance of the multiple sclerosis functional composite: relationship to patient-reported quality of life 12. Arch Neurol 2000;57(9):1319–1324.

36. Janardhan V, Bakshi R. Quality of life and its relationship to brain lesions and atrophy on magnetic resonance images in 60 patients with multiple sclerosis. Arch Neurol 2000;57(10): 1485–1491.

37. Benito-Leon J, Morales JM, Rivera-Navarro J. Health-related quality of life and its relationship to cognitive and emotional functioning in multi-ple sclerosis patients. Eur J Neurol 2002;9(5):497–502.

38. Shawaryn MA, Schiaffino KM, LaRocca NG, Johnston MV. Determinants of health-related quality of life in multiple sclerosis: the role of illness intrusiveness. Mult Scler 2002;8(4):310–318.

39. Rao SM, Hammeke TA, McQuillen MP, Khatri BO, Lloyd D. Memory disturbance in chronic progressive multiple sclerosis. Arch Neurol 1984;41(6):625–631.

40. Rao SM, Leo GJ, Ellington L, et al. Cognitive dysfunction in multiple sclerosis. II. Impact on employment and social functioning. Neurology 1991;41(5):692–696.

41. Thornton AE, Raz N. Memory impairment in multiple sclerosis: a quantitative review. Neuropsychology 1997;11(3):357–366.

42. McIntosh-Michaelis SA, Roberts MH, Wilkinson SM, et al. The prevalence of cognitive impairment in a community survey of multiple sclerosis. Br J Clin Psychol 1991;30(Pt 4):333–348.

43. Minden SL, Moes EJ, Orav J, Kaplan E, Reich P. Memory impairment in multiple sclerosis. J Clin Exp Neuropsychol 1990;12(4):566–586.

44. Heaton RK, Nelson LM, Thompson DS, Burks JS, Franklin GM. Neuropsychological findings in relapsing-remitting and chronic-progressive multiple sclerosis. J Consult Clin Psychol 1985;53(1):103–110.

45. Chelune GJ, Stone L. Relative risk of cognitive impairment is mediated by disease course and sex in multiple sclerosis. International Neuropsychological Society, 33rd Annual Meeting, 2005:42–43.

46. Gaudino EA, Chiaravalloti ND, DeLuca J, Diamond BJ. A comparison of memory performance in relapsing-remitting, primary progressive and secondary progressive, multiple sclerosis. Neuropsychiatry Neuropsychol Behav Neurol 2001; 14(1):32–44.

47. Gonzalez CF, Swirsky-Sacchetti T, Mitchell D, et al. Distributional patterns of multiple sclerosis brain lesions. Magnetic resonance imaging – clinical correlation. J Neuroimaging 1994;4(4):188–195.

48. Comi G, Filippi M, Martinelli V, et al. Brain MRI correlates of cognitive impairment in primary and secondary progressive multiple sclerosis 2114. J Neurol Sci 1995;132(2): 222–227.

49. Beatty WW, Aupperle RL. Sex differences in cognitive impairment in multiple sclerosis. Clin Neuropsychol 2002;16(4):472–480.

50. Beatty WW, Goodkin DE, Hertsgaard D, Monson N. Clinical and demographic predictors of cognitive performance in multiple sclerosis. Do diagnostic type, disease duration, and disability matter? Arch Neurol 1990;47(3):305–308.

51. Krupp LB, Elkins LE. Fatigue and declines in cognitive functioning in multiple sclerosis. Neurology 2000;55(7):934–939.

52. Schwid SR, Tyler CM, Scheid EA, et al. Cognitive fatigue during a test requiring sustained attention: a pilot study. Mult Scler 2003;9(5):503–508.

53. Parmenter BA, Denney DR, Lynch SG. The cognitive performance of patients with multiple sclerosis during periods of high and low fatigue. Mult Scler 2003;9(2):111–118.

54. Beatty WW, Goretti B, Siracusa G, et al. Changes in neuropsychological test performance over the workday in multiple sclerosis. Clin Neuropsychol 2003;17:551–560.

55. Feinstein A. The neuropsychiatry of multiple sclerosis. Can J Psychiatry 2004;49:157–163.

56. Benedict RH, Priore RL, Miller C, Munschauer F, Jacobs L. Personality disorder in multiple sclerosis correlates with cognitive impairment. J Neuropsychiatry Clin Neurosci 2001;13(1):70–76.

57. Feinstein A, Feinstein K, Gray T, O'Connor P. Prevalence and neurobehavioral correlates of pathological laughing and crying in multiple sclerosis. Arch Neurol 1997;54(9): 1116–1121.

58. Arnett PA, Higginson CI, Randolph JJ. Depression in multiple sclerosis: relationship to planning ability. J Int Neuropsychol Soc 2001;7(6): 665–674.

59. Arnett PA, Higginson CI, Voss WD, Randolph JJ, Grandey AA. Relationship between coping, cognitive dysfunction and depression in multiple sclerosis. Clin Neuropsychol 2002;16(3):341–355.

60. Sperling RA, Guttmann CR, Hohol MJ, et al. Regional magnetic resonance imaging lesion burden and cognitive function in multiple sclerosis: a longitudinal study. Arch Neurol 2001;58(1):115–121.

61. Bermel RA, Bakshi R, Tjoa C, Puli SR, Jacobs L. Bicaudate ratio as a magnetic resonance imaging marker of brain atrophy in multiple sclerosis. Arch Neurol 2002;59(2):275–280.

62. Benedict RH, Weinstock-Guttman B, Fishman I, et al. Prediction of neuropsychological impairment in multiple sclerosis: comparison of conventional magnetic resonance imaging measures of atrophy and lesion burden. Arch Neurol 2004; 61(2):226–230.

63. Edwards SG, Liu C, Blumhardt LD. Cognitive correlates of supratentorial atrophy on MRI in multiple sclerosis. Acta Neurol Scand 2001;104(4): 214–223.

64. Benedict RH, Bakshi R, Simon JH, et al. Frontal cortex atrophy predicts cognitive impairment in multiple sclerosis. J Neuropsychiatry Clin Neurosci 2002;14(1):44–51.

65. Carone D, Zivadinov R, Weinstock-Guttman B, et al. Learning inconsistency is associated with frontal lobe atrophy in multiple sclerosis.

International Neuropsychological Society, 33rd Annual Meeting, 2005:42.

66. Nocentini U, Rossini PM, Carlesimo GA, et al. Patterns of cognitive impairment in secondary progressive stable phase of multiple sclerosis: correlations with MRI findings. Eur Neurol 2001;45(1):11–18.

67. Rocca MA, Pagani E, Ghezzi A, et al. Functional cortical changes in patients with multiple sclerosis and nonspecific findings on conventional magnetic resonance imaging scans of the brain. Neuroimage 2003;19(3): 826–836.

68. Rocca MA, Gavazzi C, Mezzapesa DM, et al. A functional magnetic resonance imaging study of patients with secondary progressive multiple sclerosis. Neuroimage 2003;19(4): 1770–1777.

69. Filippi M, Rocca MA, Falini A, et al. Correlations between structural CNS damage and functional MRI changes in primary progressive MS. Neuroimage 2002;15(3):537–546.

70. Pozzilli C, Passafiume D, Bernardi S, et al. SPECT, MRI and cognitive functions in multiple sclerosis. J Neurol Neurosurg Psychiatry 1991;54(2):110–115.

71. Pantano P, Mainero C, Iannetti GD, et al. Contribution of corticospinal tract damage to cortical motor reorganization after a single clinical attack of multiple sclerosis. Neuroimage 2002; 17:1837–1843.

72. Reddy H, Narayanan S, Woolrich M, et al. Functional brain reorganization for hand movement in patients with multiple sclerosis: defining distinct effects of injury and disability. Brain 2002;125(Pt 12):2646–2657.

73. Filippi M, Rocca MA, Colombo B, et al. Functional magnetic resonance imaging correlates of fatigue in multiple sclerosis. Neuroimage 2002; 15(3):559–567.

74. Rocca MA, Mezzapesa DM, Falini A, et al. Evidence for axonal pathology and adaptive cortical reorganization in patients at presentation with clinically isolated syndromes suggestive of multiple sclerosis. Neuroimage 2003;18(4):847–855.

75. Staffen W, Mair A, Zauner H,et al. Cognitive function and fMRI in patients with multiple sclerosis: evidence for compensatory cortical activation during an attention task. Brain 2002;125(Pt6):1275–1282.

76. Mainero C, Caramia F, Pozzilli C, et al. fMRI evidence of brain reorganization during attention and memory tasks in multiple sclerosis. Neuroimage 2004;21(3):858–867.

77. Audoin B, Ibarrola D, Ranjeva JP, et al. Compensatory cortical activation observed by fMRI during a cognitive task at the earliest stage of MS. Hum Brain Mapp 2003;20(2):51–58.

78. Hillary FG, Chiaravalloti ND, Ricker JH, et al. An investigation of working memory rehearsal in multiple sclerosis using fMRI. J Clin Exp Neuropsychol 2003;25(7):965–978.

79. Sweet LH, Paul RH, Cohen RA, et al. Neuroimaging correlates of dementia rating scale performance at baseline and 12-month follow-up among patients with vascular dementia. J Geriatr Psychiatry Neurol 2003; 16(4):240–244.

80. Wishart HA, Saykin AJ, McDonald BC, et al. Brain activation patterns associated with working memory in relapsing-remitting MS. Neurology 2004; 62(2):234–238.

81. Li Y, Chiaravalloti ND, Hillary FG, et al. Differential cerebellar activation on functional magnetic resonance imaging during working memory performance in persons with multiple sclerosis. Arch Phys Med Rehabil 2004;85:635–639.

82. Lazeron RH, Rombouts SA, Scheltens P, Polman C, Barkhof F. An fMRI study of planning-related brain activity in patients with moderately advanced multiple sclerosis. Mult Scler 2004;10:549–555.

83. Parry AM, Scott RB, Palace J, Smith S, Matthews PM. Potentially adaptive functional changes in cognitive processing for patients with multiple sclerosis and their acute modulation by rivastigmine. Brain 2003;126(Pt 12):2750–2760.

84. Amato MP, Zipoli V. Clinical management of cognitive impairment in multiple sclerosis: a review of current evidence. Int MS J 2003;10(3):72–83.

85. Fischer JS, Priore RL, Jacobs LD, et al. Neuropsychological effects of interferon beta-1a in relapsing multiple sclerosis. Multiple Sclerosis Collaborative Research Group. Ann Neurol 2000;48(6):885–892.

86. Barak Y, Achiron A. Effect of interferon-beta-1b on cognitive functions in multiple sclerosis. Eur Neurol 2002;47(1):11–14.

87. Pliskin NH, Hamer DP, Goldstein DS, et al. Improved delayed visual reproduction test performance in multiple sclerosis patients receiving interferon beta-1b. Neurology 1996; 47(6):1463–1468.

88. Selby MJ, Ling N, Williams JM, Dawson A. Interferon beta 1-b in verbal memory functioning of patients with relapsing-remitting multiple sclerosis. Percept Mot Skills 1998; 86(3 Pt 1):1099–1106.

89. Weinstein A, Schwid SI, Schiffer RB, et al. Neuropsychologic status in multiple sclerosis after treatment with glatiramer. Arch Neurol 1999;56(3):319–324.

90. Greene YM, Tariot PN, Wishart H, et al. A 12-week, open trial of donepezil hydrochloride in patients with multiple sclerosis and associated cognitive impairments. J Clin Psychopharmacol 2000;20(3):350–356.

91. Krupp LB, Elkins LE, Scheffer RS, Smiroldo J, Coyle P. Donepezil for the treatment of memory impairment in multiple sclerosis. Neurology 1999;52:A137.

92. Krupp LB, Christodoulou C, Melville P, et al. Donepezil improved memory in multiple sclerosis in a randomized clinical trial. Neurology 2004;63: 1579–1585.

93. Cohen RA, Fischer M. Amantadine treatment of fatigue associated with multiple sclerosis. Arch Neurol 1989; 46:676–680.

94. Geisler MW, Sliwinski M, Coyle PK, et al. The effects of amantadine and pemoline on cognitive functioning in multiple sclerosis. Arch Neurol 1996;53(2):185–188.

95. Patzold T, Schwengelbeck M, Ossege LM, Malin JP, Sindern E. Changes of the MS functional composite and EDSS during and after treatment of relapses with methylprednisolone in patients with multiple sclerosis. Acta Neurol Scand 2002;105(3):164–168.

96. Gillson G, Richard TL, Smith RB, Wright JV. A double-blind pilot study of the effect of Prokarin on fatigue in multiple sclerosis. Mult Scler 2002; 8(1):30–35.

97. Rossini PM, Pasqualetti P, Pozzilli C, et al. Fatigue in progressive multiple sclerosis: results of a randomized, double-blind, placebo-controlled, crossover trial of oral 4-aminopyridine. Mult Scler 2001; 7(6):354–358.

98. Mohr DC, Cox D. Multiple sclerosis: empirical literature for the clinical health psychologist. J Clin Psychol 2001;57(4):479–499.

99. Allen DN, Goldstein G, Heyman RA, Rondinelli T. Teaching memory strategies to persons with multiple sclerosis. J Rehabil Res Dev 1998; 35:405–410.

100. Canellopoulou M, Richardson JT. The role of executive function in imagery mnemonics: evidence from multiple sclerosis. Neuropsychologia 1998;36(11):1181–1188.

101. Jonsson A, Korfitzen EM, Heltberg A, Ravnborg MH, Byskov-Ottosen E. Effects of neuropsychological treatment in patients with multiple sclerosis. Acta Neurol Scand 1993; 88(6):394–400.

102. Mendozzi L, Pugnetti L. Computer assisted memory retraining of patients with multiple sclerosis. Ital J Neurol Sci 1998;19:S431–S438.

103. Plohmann A, Kappos L, Ammann W, et al. Computer assisted retraining of attentional impairments in patients with multiple sclerosis. J Neurol Neurosurg Psychiatry 1998;64: 455–462.

104. Rodgers D, Khoo K, MacEachen M, Oven M, Beatty WW. Cognitive therapy for multiple sclerosis: a preliminary study. Altern Ther Health Med 1996;2(5):70–74.

105. Benedict RH, Shapiro A, Priore R, et al. Neuropsychological counseling improves social behavior in cognitively-impaired multiple sclerosis patients. Mult Scler 2000;6(6): 391–396.

11

Cholinesterase inhibitors in the treatment of dementia associated with Parkinson's disease

Murat Emre

INTRODUCTION

Parkinson's disease (PD), the second most frequent neurodegenerative disorder after Alzheimer's disease (AD), has been accepted to be mainly a disorder of the motor system for many years. This was probably because of the original description, i.e. that senses and intellect remain intact, but also probably because the patients did not survive long enough in the initial decades following the description of the disease. As more effective treatments became available and survival time for PD patients became longer, cognitive deficits and dementia associated with PD (PD-D) have become increasingly more recognized. We now understand that subtle cognitive deficits are already present in newly diagnosed patient populations;[1] dementia is a frequently encountered and a markedly age-dependent phenomenon among patients with PD. A meta-analysis of cross-sectional studies revealed a frequency of 40%,[2] whereas prospective observational studies suggest that as many as 78% of patients may become affected by dementia as the age and disease severity progress.[3] Remarkable is the effect of age: in a population-based study, the prevalence of dementia below 50 years old was found to be 0%; above 80 years old, it reached 69%.[4] It seems that the combined effect of advanced age and severe disease is detrimental: in an observational study, old patients with severe disease at baseline had a 9.7-fold increase in incident dementia as compared to young patients with mild disease.[5]

In the last two decades neuropathology and neurochemical deficits accompanying PD-D have been increasingly better understood. Morphologic and biochemical studies have revealed prominent cholinergic deficits associated with PD-D. As cholinergic treatment with choline esterase inhibitors (ChE-Is) became available and widely administered in AD, these drugs were also investigated in PD-D. This chapter summarizes the cholinergic deficits found in patients with PD-D and the results of treatment attempts with ChE-Is.

CHOLINERGIC DEFICITS IN DEMENTIA ASSOCIATED WITH PARKINSON'S DISEASE

Cholinergic deficits in PD-D were reported shortly after they were described in AD, and they were then confirmed in subsequent studies. These included decrease in the number of cholinergic cells in the basal forebrain cholinergic nuclei, decrease in the amount of cortical cholinergic markers, both biochemically and in in-vivo imaging studies, and evidence for functional deficits.

Cholinergic cell loss

Loss of cholinergic cells in the nucleus basalis of Meynert (nbM) in patients with PD-D were described by Whitehouse et al in 1983.[6] In parallel, Candy et al described that neuronal loss from the nBM was greater in patients with PD than those with AD.[7] Shortly thereafter, Nakano and Hirano described that nbM was significantly depleted of its large neurons in Parkinson's disease and that this loss was not associated with AD-type pathology in the cerebral cortex.[8]

Biochemical findings

In parallel to the morphologic findings, biochemical deficits in nbM and in cerebral cortex were described, beginning from the early 1980s. Thus, choline acetyltransferase (ChAT) activity was found to be decreased in the frontal cortex and nbM of patients with PD, the decrease being greater in the frontal cortex of PD patients with dementia.[9] Similarly Perry et al[10] described that in PD patients with dementia there were extensive reductions of ChAT and less extensive reductions of acetylcholinesterase (AChE) in all examined cortical areas from four different cerebral lobes, and ChAT reductions in temporal neocortex correlated with the degree of mental impairment but not with the extent of plaque or tangle formation. In addition, in PD but not in AD, the decrease in neocortical ChAT levels correlated with the number of neurons in nbM, suggesting that primary degeneration of these cholinergic neurons may be related to declining cognitive function in PD.[10] In a comparative study with AD, the same group of researchers reported that amongst the various pathologic and chemical indices examined, only presynaptic cholinergic markers (including the number of neurons in nbM) and serotonin S1-receptor binding were related to dementia in PD.[11] They also reported that reductions in ChAT activity were generally more extensive in the neocortical (especially temporal) as opposed to archicortical regions, nicotinic receptor binding in cortex was reduced, and muscarinic binding was increased.[12,13] A relevant finding was that nicotinic receptor binding was also reduced in striatum in patients with PD, suggesting a reduced risk of parkinsonism with AChE-I through stimulation of striatal cholinergic receptors.[14] Finally, in a comparative study of patients with AD, DLB (LB variant and Diffuse Lewy Body Disease) and PD, mean midfrontal ChAT activity was found to be markedly reduced in PD and DLB compared with normal controls and AD: the activity was reduced to almost 20% of controls in DLB and PD, whereas in AD it was reduced to 50% of the activity in normals.[15]

In-vivo and functional deficits

Reductions in cortical cholinergic activity in patients with PD-D were also demonstrated in vivo, and clinical studies suggested subtle, subclinical deficits already in non-demented patients. In a double-blind cross-over study, Dubois et al[16] compared the effects of a subthreshold dose of scopolamine on memory in 32 control subjects and 32 PD patients who had no signs of intellectual or memory impairment. Controls showed no impairment of memory after scopolamine, whereas the same dose resulted in a significant reduction of memory performance involving visual recognition. This selective vulnerability in patients without apparent cognitive impairment, to a subthreshold dose of scopolamine, suggested the existence of an underlying deficit in central cholinergic transmission.[16] The same group of investigators,[17] subsequently reported that, as compared to patients who were matched for all the variables of parkinsonism and levodopa therapy, but not receiving anticholinergics, PD patients who were on anticholinergics performed significantly worse in tests believed to assess frontal lobe function, whereas there was no significant difference between the two groups for intellectual, visuospatial, instrumental, and memory functions. The authors suggested that impairment in ascending cholinergic activity may play a role in the impairment of functions subserved by subcortical-frontal circuits in these patients.[17] Recently, in-vivo imaging of cortical cholinergic function using positron emission tomography (PET) revealed that, compared with controls, mean cortical AChE activity was lowest in patients with PD-D (−20%), followed by patients with PD without dementia (−13%) and AD (−9%). Thus, reduced cortical AChE activity seemed to be more characteristic of patients with PD-D than of patients with mild AD, both groups having similar severity of dementia.[18]

EFFECTS OF CHOLINESTERASE INHIBITORS ON DEMENTIA ASSOCIATED WITH PARKINSON'S DISEASE

Although cholinergic deficits accompanying PD-D were described shortly after those accompanying AD and cholinergic treatment strategies, i.e. ChE-Is became widely available for treatment of AD, there was an initial hesitation to use them in PD-D because of the fear that motor functions may be worsened, due to the disturbed dopaminergic/cholinergic balance in PD, in favor of the latter. These fears were partly overcome by an initial study with tacrine that described rather dramatic improvements and no worsening in motor functions in patients with PD and cognitive impairment.[19] Since then, a number of studies have been reported with all commercially available ChE-I. These studies are summarized in Table 11.1

Tacrine

Seven PD patients with cognitive impairment and psychotic symptoms were treated with tacrine over eight weeks in an open-label study.[19] Rather dramatic improvements were reported; importantly, motor symptoms did not seem to worsen and a few patients even showed improvement in their motor function. The dramatic beneficial response described in this study was not replicated to the same extent; nevertheless, this was an important study that paved the way for further trials. In another study, 7 out of 11 patients were treated with tacrine and 4 with donepezil over 26 weeks in an open-label fashion. Patients under both treatments showed improvement in their cognitive functions, there was no deterioration in motor scores, and 5 patients even demonstrated some motor improvement.[20]

Table 11.1	List of studies with cholinesterase inhibitors in dementia associated with Parkinson's disease		
Reference	*n*	Design	Treatment duration (weeks)
Tacrine			
Hutchinson 1996[19]	7	Open	8
Werber 2001[20]	7/11	Open	26
Donepezil			
Aarsland 2002[25]	14	RCT cross-over	10+10
Bergman 2002[22]	6	Open	6
Fabbrini 2002[23]	8	Open	8
Minett 2003[24]	15	Open treat/withdraw/treat/	20/6/12
Kurita 2003[21]	3	Chart review	2–52
Leroi 2004[26]	16	RCT	18
Brashear 2004[27]	20	RCT	12+33 (OL)
Rivastigmine			
Reading 2001[30]	15	Open/washout	14/3
Bullock 2002[29]	5	Chart review	20–52
Giladi 2003[31]	28	Open/washout	26/8
Emre 2004[32]	541	RCT	26
Galantamine			
Aarsland 2003[28]	16	Open	8
RCT = randomized controlled trial; OL = open label.			

Donepezil

There have been seven reported studies with donepezil in patients with PD and either dementia, or cognitive impairment, or psychotic symptoms such as visual hallucinations and delusions. One of the studies was a small case series of 3 patients, describing improvement in visual hallucinations;[21] three of the studies were open studies with small numbers; and three of the studies were small, randomized, placebo-controlled studies, either with a parallel group or cross-over design. In the open studies, which included 6–15 patients and lasted 6–20 weeks, psychotic features, including visual hallucinations, improved in all patients and cognitive function, as measured with the MMSE (Mini-Mental State Examination), was reported to improve in one study and remained unchanged in the other two studies. Motor symptoms seemed to be unaffected in two studies, but worsening was reported in 2 out of 8 patients in the third study.[22–24] One study suggested that hallucinations consistently improved on treatment and worsened after withdrawal; the authors recommended avoiding an abrupt withdrawal of medication, which may produce acute cognitive and behavioral decline.[24]

The three randomized controlled studies with donepezil involved 14–23 patients and treatment duration was 10–18 weeks; one of the studies included a 33-week open-label extension period.[25–27] In all three studies, there was an improvement in cognitive functions, mostly on MMSE. Visual hallucinations were assessed only in one study and were not improved. Motor symptoms did not worsen in two studies and in the double-blind phase of the third study, but during the open-label extension of the latter there seemed to be a deterioration of motor function, UPDRS (Unified Parkinson's Disease Rating Scale) total and subscores were worse than baseline, and 8 out of the 15 patients remaining in the extension phase reported worsening of parkinsonism.[27]

Galantamine

There has been only one reported study with galantamine in patients with PD-D. In this open-label study, 16 patients were treated with galantamine over 8 weeks. 'Global mental functions' improved in 8 and worsened in 4 patients; tests such as MMSE, clock drawing, and verbal fluency showed improvements that favored galantamine. Hallucinations improved in 7 out of 9 patients who had hallucinations at baseline. Parkinsonism, as assessed clinically, was reported to be improved in 6 patients; however, a mild worsening of tremor was observed in 3 patients.[28]

Rivastigmine

There have been three earlier reports of rivastigmine use in PD-D. One study, a case series involving 5 patients which reported improvement in cognitive and functional abilities as well as resolution of behavioral problems such as visual hallucinations.[29] The other two[30,31] were open label studies that comprised 15 and 28 patients, and the duration of treatment was 14 and 26 weeks, respectively. In both studies, cognitive functions, as measured by MMSE in one and in addition with ADAS-cog (Alzheimer's Disease Assessment Scale – Cognitive) and CGI (Clinical Global Impression) in the other, significantly improved from baseline. Visual hallucinations were assessed only in one study and showed significant improvements. In both studies there was no worsening of motor symptoms.[30,31]

Recently, the first large, randomized, controlled, multicenter study ever conducted with a ChE-I in PD-D was published.[32] This study, known as EXPRESS, included 68 centers from 12 countries. Altogether, 541 patients with a diagnosis of PD, according to UK Brain Bank criteria, and dementia due to PD, according to DSM IV (Diagnostic and Statistical Manual of Mental Disorders – 4th edn), were randomized to rivastigmine or placebo with a ratio of 2:1. In order to differentiate from patients fulfilling the current criteria for DLB, patients were required to have at least 2 years' interval between the onset of their motor and cognitive symptoms. Patients with exposure to ChE-I or anticholinergics within the last 3 months before entry into the study and patients with evidence for other neurodegenerative disorders or any unstable systemic disease were excluded. Primary efficacy parameters included ADAS-cog for cognitive functions and ADCS-CGIC (Alzheimer's Disease Cooperative Study – Clinical Global Impression of Change Scale) for global assessment of change in the overall status of patients. Secondary clinical efficacy parameters included MMSE for screening and staging, ADCS-ADL (Alzheimer's Disease Cooperative Study – Activities of Daily Living) for the assessment of daily living, NPI (Neuropsychiatric Inventory) for the assessment of neuropsychiatric symptoms, a computerized test battery for the assessment of attention (Clinical Dementia Rating (CDR) power of attention tests), and two tests for the assessment of executive functions including verbal fluency from D-KEFS (Delis–Kaplan Executive Function System) test battery and Ten-Point Clock Drawing Test. Safety parameters included recording of adverse events, laboratory evaluations, vital signs including pulse, blood pressure and body weight, ECG (electro-cardiography) and UPDRS Part III for the assessment of motor functions.

Out of the 541 patients entered in the study, 410 completed and 131 patients prematurely discontinued. Discontinuations were more in the rivastigmine group (27.3% vs 17.9% under placebo); this was also the case for discontinuations because of adverse events (17.1% vs 7.8% under placebo); Both primary efficacy endpoints showed statistically significant improvements in favor of rivastigmine. On ADAS-cog, patients on rivastigmine showed a 2.1 improvement at 26 weeks, from a baseline value of 23.8, whereas patients on placebo deteriorated by 0.7 points (from a baseline score of 24.3), yielding a 2.9 points or 11.7% treatment difference from baseline ($p < 0.001$). The mean scores for the ADCS-CGIC at week 24 were 3.8 in the rivastigmine and 4.3 in the placebo group (score 4 indicating no change, lower scores indicating improvement, and higher scores indicating worsening from baseline);

comparison of outcomes across all response categories revealed a statistically significant difference in favor of rivastigmine ($p = 0.007$). More patients on rivastigmine improved (40.8% vs 29.7% on placebo) and more patients on placebo deteriorated (42.5% on placebo vs 33.7% on rivastigmine). Considering the number of patients who had a clinically relevant change (marked or moderate change), a similar picture emerged: 19.8.% of patients had marked or moderate improvement on rivastigmine vs 14.5% of patients on placebo, whereas 23.1% of patients had marked or moderate worsening on placebo vs 13% on rivastigmine. On all secondary efficacy parameters, there were statistically significant differences in favor of rivastigmine. Thus, neuropsychiatric symptoms, as measured with NPI, showed an improvement on rivastigmine and no change from baseline on placebo, power of attention improved on rivastigmine and worsened on placebo, and improvement from baseline was also seen on the Ten-Point Clock Drawing test, verbal fluency, and MMSE on rivastigmine, whereas patients on placebo worsened as compared with baseline scores. On ADCS-ADL, patients on rivastigmine showed a minimal worsening, whereas patients on placebo had significantly more deterioration (Table 11.2).

Adverse events were significantly more frequent on rivastigmine. Main adverse events were those related to the gastrointestinal system – nausea and vomiting being the most frequent ones (29.0% vs 11.2% nausea, and 16.6 % vs 1.7% vomiting on rivastigmine and placebo, respectively). Worsening of parkinsonian symptoms was more frequently reported as an adverse event on rivastigmine (27.3% vs 15.6% on placebo), mainly driven by worsening of tremor (10.2% on rivastigmine vs 3.9% on placebo). The objective measures of motor symptoms, however, as assessed by UPDRS part III did not reveal any

Table 11.2 Primary and secondary efficacy parameters in the EXPRESS study[a]

Scale	Rivastigmine	Placebo	p-value
Primary			
ADAS-cog	2.1	−0.7	< 0.001
ADCS-CGIC	3.8	4.3	0.007
Secondary			
ADCS-ADL	−1.1	−3.6	0.02
NPI	2.0	0.0	0.02
CDR power of attention	31.0	−142.7	0.009
MMSE	0.8	−0.2	0.03
Verbal fluency	1.7	−1.1	< 0.001
Ten-Point Clock Drawing	0.5	−0.6	0.02

[a] The numbers indicate changes from baseline at week 26. For ease of understanding, improvements from baseline are shown as positive, and deteriorations as negative values, except for ADCS-CGIC, for which there was no baseline value, as this scale itself assesses change from baseline. For ADCS-CGIC, scores below 4 indicate improvement and above 4 indicate worsening. For written-out versions of scales, see text (Emre et al, 2004).

significant differences or trends between the two treatments. There were no clinically relevant changes on vital signs, body weight, ECG, or laboratory parameters.

CONCLUSIONS

Parkinson's disease is frequently associated with dementia: up to 40% of patients with PD may be affected, especially at higher ages and in the later stages of the disease. There are prominent cholinergic deficits accompanying dementia associated with PD. A number of small, mostly open studies with all available ChE-Is and one large, randomized, controlled study with rivastigmine revealed beneficial effects of ChE-Is in these patients. The large, randomized, placebo-controlled EXPRESS study demonstrated that rivastigmine improves deficits in all key symptom domains, including cognitive dysfunction and behavioral symptoms; these benefits are reflected in the overall status and functioning of patients. This study also revealed that there was no worsening of motor functions under rivastigmine, except for 10% of patients reporting a worsening of their tremor as an adverse event. Taking together all the available evidence, especially the results of the EXPRESS study with rivastigmine, it can be concluded that ChE-Is represent an effective approach in the treatment of dementia associated with PD.

REFERENCES

1. Foltynie T, Brayne CEG, Robbins TW, Barker RA. The cognitive ability of an incident cohort of Parkinson's patients in the UK. The CamPaIGN study. Brain 2004;127(Pt 3):550–560.

2. Cummings JL. Intellectual impairment in Parkinson's disease: clinical, pathologic, and biochemical correlates. J Geriatr Psychiatry Neurol 1988;1(1):24–36.

3. Aarsland D, Andersen K, Larsen JP, et al. Prevalence and characteristics of dementia in Parkinson disease: an 8-year prospective study. Arch Neurol 2003;60(3):387–392.

4. Mayeux R, Denaro J, Hemenegildo N, et al. A population-based investigation of Parkinson's disease with and without dementia. Relationship to age and gender. Arch Neurol 1992; 49(5):492–497.

5. Levy G, Schupf N, Tang MX, et al. Combined effect of age and severity on the risk of dementia in Parkinson's disease. Ann Neurol 2002;51(6):722–729.

6. Whitehouse PJ, Hedreen JC, White CL 3rd, Price DL. Basal forebrain neurons in the dementia of Parkinson disease. Ann Neurol 1983; 13:243–248.

7. Candy JM, Perry RH, Perry EK, et al. Pathological changes in the nucleus of Meynert in Alzheimer's and Parkinson's diseases. J Neurol Sci 1983;59:277–289.

8. Nakano I, Hirano A. Parkinson's disease: neuron loss in the nucleus basalis without concomitant Alzheimer's disease. Ann Neurol 1984;15:415–418.

9. Dubois B, Ruberg M, Javoy-Agid F, Ploska A, Agid Y. A subcortico-cortical cholinergic system is affected in Parkinson's disease. Brain Res 1983;288:213–218.

10. Perry EK, Curtis M, Dick DJ, et al. Cholinergic correlates of cognitive impairment in Parkinson's disease: comparisons with Alzheimer's disease. J Neurol Neurosurg Psychiatry 1985;48:413–421.

11. Perry RH, Perry EK, Smith CJ, et al. Cortical neuropathological and neurochemical substrates of Alzheimer's and Parkinson's diseases. J Neural Transm Suppl 1987;24:131–136.

12. Perry EK, Smith CJ, Court JA, Perry RH. Cholinergic nicotinic and muscarinic receptors in dementia of Alzheimer, Parkinson and Lewy body types. J Neural Transm Park Dis Dement Sect 1990;2:149–158.

13. Perry EK, Irving D, Kerwin JM, et al. Cholinergic transmitter and neurotrophic activities in Lewy body dementia: similarity to Parkinson's and distinction from Alzheimer disease. Alzheimer Dis Assoc Disord 1993;7:69–79.

14. Pimlott SL, Piggott M, Owens J, et al. Nicotinic acetylcholine receptor distribution in Alzheimer's disease, dementia with Lewy bodies, Parkinson's disease, and vascular dementia: in vitro binding study using 5-[(125)i]-a-85380. Neuropsychopharmacology 2004;29:108–116.

15. Tiraboschi P, Hansen LA, Alford M, et al. Cholinergic dysfunction in diseases with Lewy bodies. Neurology 2000;54:407–411.

16. Dubois B, Danze F, Pillon B, et al. Cholinergic-dependent cognitive deficits in Parkinson's disease. Ann Neurol 1987;22:26–30.

17. Dubois B, Pilon B, Lhermitte F, Agid Y. Cholinergic deficiency and frontal dysfunction in Parkinson's disease. Ann Neurol 1990;28:117–121.

18. Bohnen NI, Kaufer DI, Ivanco LS, et al. Cortical cholinergic function is more severely affected in parkinsonian dementia than in Alzheimer disease: an in vivo positron emission tomographic study. Arch Neurol 2003;60:1745–1748.

19. Hutchinson M, Fazzini E. Cholinesterase inhibition in Parkinson's disease. J Neurol Neurosurg Psychiatry 1996;61(3):324–325.

20. Werber EA, Rabey JM. The beneficial effect of cholinesterase inhibitors on patients suffering from Parkinson's disease and dementia. J Neural Transm 2001;108(11):1319–1325.

21. Kurita A, Ochiai Y, Kono Y, Suzuki M, Inoue K. The beneficial effect of donepezil on visual hallucinations in three patients with Parkinson's disease. J Geriatr Psychiatry Neurol 2003; 6(3):184–188.

22. Bergman J, Lerner V. Successful use of donepezil for the treatment of psychotic symptoms in patients with Parkinson's disease. Clin Neuropharmacol 2002;25:107–110.

23. Fabbrini G, Barbanti P, Aurilia C, et al. Donepezil in the treatment of hallucinations and delusions in Parkinson's disease. Neurol Sci 2002;23:41–43.

24. Minett TS, Thomas A, Wilkinson LM, et al. What happens when donepezil is suddenly withdrawn? An open label trial in dementia with Lewy bodies and Parkinson's disease with dementia. Int J Geriatr Psychiatry 2003;18(11):988–993

25. Aarsland D, Laake K, Larsen JP, Janvin C. Donepezil for cognitive impairment in Parkinson's disease: a randomised controlled study. J Neurol Neurosurg Psychiatry 2002; 72:708–712.

26. Leroi I, Brandt J, Reich SG, et al. Randomized placebo-controlled trial of donepezil in cognitive impairment in Parkinson's disease. Int J Geriatr Psychiatry 2004;19:1–8.

27. Brashear A, Kuhn ER, Lane KA, Farlow MR, Unverzagt FW. A dou-

ble-blind, placebo-controlled trial of donepezil in patients with Parkinson's disease and related dementia. Neurology 2004;62(Suppl 5):524.

28. Aarsland D, Hutchinson M, Larsen JP. Cognitive, psychiatric and motor response to galantamine in Parkinson's disease with dementia. Int J Geriatr Psychiatry 2003; 18:937–941.

29. Bullock R, Cameron A. Rivastigmine for the treatment of dementia and visual hallucinations associated with Parkinson's disease: a case series. Curr Med Res Opin 2002; 18:258–264.

30. Reading PJ, Luce AK, McKeith IG. Rivastigmine in the treatment of parkinsonian psychosis and cognitive impairment: preliminary findings from an open trial. Mov Disord 2001; 16:1171–1174.

31. Giladi N, Shabtai H, Benbunan B, et al. The effect of treatment with rivastigmine (Exelon) on cognitive functions of patients with dementia and Parkinson's disease. Acta Neurol Scand 2003;108(5):368–373.

32. Emre M, Aarsland D, Albanese A, et al. Rivastigmine for dementia associated with Parkinson's disease. N Engl J Med 2004;351:2509–2518.

12

Modern applications of electroencephalography in dementia diagnosis*

CJ Stam

INTRODUCTION

What use is electroencephalography (EEG) in the diagnosis of dementia? This question seems deceptively simple, but despite many years of research and hundreds of papers published on this topic the role of the EEG in the diagnosis and assessment of dementia is still controversial. The widely differing opinions on the usefulness of the EEG in dementia are reflected in the way the EEG is dealt with in the various consensus texts on dementia diagnosis. For instance, while a Scandinavian consensus text recommends to record an EEG in all subjects with suspected dementia, the US text does not even mention EEG as a possible laboratory test.[1,2] Given this lack of consensus and the enormous and rapidly growing literature on the topic, the clinician is faced with the difficult questions of whether the EEG will be of any use in assessing patients who present with cognitive complaints and what is the optimal way to use the EEG in this category of patients. This chapter is intended to address this question, and to suggest a practical approach to the use of EEG in dementia diagnosis. First, EEG findings in normal aging and various types of dementia are discussed. Next, a practical approach to EEG diagnosis in dementia is presented. Finally, new developments and future perspectives are briefly addressed.

ELECTROENCEPHALOGRAPHIC CHANGES IN NORMAL AGING AND DEMENTIA

Normal aging

Dementia is primarily a disorder of the elderly. Therefore, EEG abnormalities in dementia have to be distinguished from physiologic EEG changes due to

*Based upon a didactic lecture presented at the 14th meeting of the European Neurological Society, Barcelona, Spain, June 2004.

normal aging.[3] Especially in the very old, this raises the question of what should be considered 'normal' or 'healthy aging'. Normal aging could be considered a statistical concept, referring to findings and characteristics in the majority of subjects in a certain age category, even when these findings might reflect subtle abnormalities. Healthy, or successful aging on the other hand, refers to optimal functioning and the absence of disease. These two different notions should be kept in mind when considering age-related EEG changes.

Aging affects physiologic EEG rhythms, most notably the alpha rhythm. The peak frequency of the alpha rhythm decreases with aging, from the normal value around 10 Hz to 8 Hz. It is unclear whether the 'normal' slowing of the alpha rhythm reflects a physiologic change in the elderly or is due to the increasing prevalence of subclinical brain disease and, in particular, dementia in this population. In clinical practice, slowing of the alpha rhythm below 8 Hz should always be considered abnormal in adult subjects at any age. Furthermore, the peak frequency in individual subjects is assumed to be fairly constant over time. Slowing of the alpha rhythm in an individual subject by more than 1 Hz is abnormal, even if the frequency is still within the normal range. Also, asymmetries of the alpha peak frequency are not a feature of normal aging but suggest brain pathology, in particular vascular disease. The reactivity of the alpha rhythm is also slightly diminished with aging. However, clear absence of reactivity to eye-opening is always abnormal. The amount of alpha activity decreases with aging, and the alpha rhythm becomes more conspicuous at posterior temporal sites and less pronounced at occipital sites.

Changes in other physiologic EEG rhythms with aging are less outspoken in the elderly. The prevalence of the mu rhythm decreases, whereas the amount of low-amplitude beta activity increases in the elderly. Activity in the theta band constitutes a special problem. In children and young subjects some amount of theta activity is normal, roughly up to an age of 25–30 years old. Interestingly, the disappearance of theta in the EEG of adults coincides with the completion of myelinization of long-range association fibers. With aging, the relative amount of theta starts to increase again. Here it is quite difficult to draw the line between normal aging and early brain pathology. This issue is further complicated by the fact that detection of moderate amounts of low-amplitude theta activity by visual analysis is difficult and unreliable. Spectral analysis of the EEG can be of some help here. As a rule of thumb, a relative theta power of more than 15% at the occipital electrodes should be considered abnormal.[4] Another possible confounding factor that should be taken into account is the influence of the level of arousal during the EEG recording. Drowsiness, which occurs rapidly and frequently during EEG recordings in the elderly and can be recognized by slow eye movements, is associated with an increase in the relative power in the theta band, especially at the central electrodes. This should not be confused with pathologic theta.

Aging is not only associated with changes in physiologic EEG rhythms but also with the emergence of new phenomena, that are assumed to have little or no pathologic meaning. The most important example of such a phenomenon is the intermittent theta and delta activity in the temporal regions, often more conspicuous on the left side. Over the age of 60 years old, such activity is found in 36% of EEG records. When the temporal theta activity fulfills certain criteria, it is designated as benign temporal theta of the elderly (BTTE) and is assumed to fall within normal limits.[3] To qualify as BTTE, the following 8 requirements have to be fulfilled:

1. the subject should be over 60 years of age;
2. the activity should be localized in the anterior temporal areas
3. the activity is more outspoken on the left side
4. the background activity should be normal
5. the amplitude should not exceed 60 μV
6. the activity should be reactive
7. the activity should occur as isolated waves and not as long trains
8. the activity should occur in less than 1% of the EEG record.

When temporal theta and delta activity does not fulfill these requirements it should be considered abnormal, and may possibly reflect vascular brain damage.

Another feature that can be seen in the EEG of healthy elderly and that can easily be mistaken for an EEG abnormality is the so-called 'sleep onset FIRDA' (frontal intermittent rhythmic delta activity). This consists of short bilaterally synchronous bursts of theta and delta which occur at transitions in the level of arousal. In contrast to the usual FIRDA, the sleep-onset FIRDA is not considered to reflect brain dysfunction. Finally, runs of sharply formed rhythmical theta activity, with a sudden start and end, can occur in the elderly without pathologic significance. These runs are indicated by the acronym SREDA (subclinical rhythmical electrical discharges of adults) and may be associated with drowsiness. SREDA should be differentiated from the rare but clinically important non-convulsive status epilepticus (sometime called 'petit mal status'), which may present as a acute confusional state and which is associated with continuous epileptic seizure activity on the EEG.[5] This is a severe condition that requires treatment with antiepileptic drugs.

Alzheimer's disease

Alzheimer's disease (AD) is the most frequent cause of dementia in the Western population. EEG changes in AD have been described in many studies over the years; reviews can be found in Boerman et al, Jonkman, and Jeong.[6–8] The changes can be characterized by the general concept of 'non-specific diffuse slowing': there is a decrease of fast frequencies (beta and alpha band) and an increase in slow frequencies (theta and delta). Loss of fast frequencies occurs relatively early, whereas the increase in delta is a relatively late phenomenon. The peak frequency of the alpha rhythm decreases, although this is not a very early finding. Increase in relative theta power may be the earliest and, from the point of view of diagnosis, the most sensitive change. Reactivity of the alpha rhythm to eye-opening also decreases, but this is difficult to quantify, and always occurs in the context of significant slowing of the background activity. Complete absence of reactivity is a rare and late finding. Intermittent slow-wave activity in the temporal regions occurs frequently in AD, but not in all patients, and may reflect concurrent vascular pathology rather than intrinsic AD pathology. Focal abnormalities and asymmetries of physiologic rhythms are not typical of AD, and may point to vascular pathology. Specific abnormalities such as sharp and triphasic waves or FIRDA occur infrequently in AD, and should always raise suspicion of metabolic or toxic encephalopathy.

Whereas slowing is the predominant feature of EEG changes in AD, another characteristic is the loss of synchronization between EEG signals recorded over different brain regions. Synchronization of EEG channels is assumed to reflect functional interactions between the underlying brain regions, and such interactions are probably affected in AD, which has been designated a 'disconnection syndrome'.[9] Functional connectivity is usually assessed by coherence analysis, which is a normalized measure of correlation between EEG channels as a function of frequency.[10] Most authors report a decrease of EEG coherence or related measures in AD, especially in the alpha band, but other bands have also been implicated.[11–21]

What causes the EEG changes in AD is not exactly known, although a few principles can be indicated. First of all, it is important to stress that the EEG does not directly reflect neuronal loss or brain atrophy. If a large number of neurons are lost, but the remaining neurons function normally, the EEG will reflect the normal function of these remaining neurons. This notion is captured by the phrase 'dead neurons tell no tales'. Consequently, the EEG abnormalities in AD and other neurodegenerative disorders must reflect abnormal functioning of the remaining neurons. There is evidence that a loss of acetylcholine, which is the most important excitatory neuromodulator in the cortex, may be responsible for the slowing of the EEG in AD.[22] Cholinergic projections to the cortex originate in the nucleus basalis of Meynert, which shows a clear loss of neurons in AD.[23] EEG slowing is related to neuron loss in the nucleus of Meynert and cholinergic deficiency in the cortex. In support of this hypothesis, treatment with drugs that activate cortical cholinergic receptors is associated with acceleration of the EEG.[24,25] This phenomenon could be used to identify patients who are more likely to respond to treatment with cholinesterase inhibitors.[26] Animal studies confirm the relationship between cholinergic deficiency to nucleus basalis lesions and EEG changes[27] and suggest that loss of cholinergic activity might also be responsible for the reduction of coherence, at least in the higher-frequency bands.[28] Disruption of interneuronal synchronization has also been ascribed directly to the amyloid plaques.[29] Some studies have attempted to relate the EEG changes in AD to the APOE genotype. The E4 allele, which is associated with an increased risk of AD, has been related to more severe EEG slowing[30] and a loss of coherence.[31] Finally, the ubiquitous loss of coherence in AD may also be due to the loss of neurons and axons connecting the involved brain areas.

Many studies have attempted to assess the diagnostic value of the EEG in AD. The reported values for the sensitivity and specificity differ widely, which may be due to differences in the populations examined (stage and severity of dementia; using healthy subjects or subjects with subjective memory complaints as controls) and differences in the various measures used to quantify the EEG abnormalities. Also, many studies involve small groups, and do not provide information on the reproducibility of the results in independent groups. Jonkman has attempted to summarize the available information, taking these limitations into account.[7] In this review, the total accuracy (percentage of correctly classified subjects) varied between 51 and 100%, with a median value of 81%. The best results are reported for slow-wave activity in REM (rapid eye movement) sleep, but this is obviously not a very practical approach.[32] On the other hand, the sensitivity of the EEG in the early stages of AD can be quite low. Up to 50% of patients with early AD may have normal EEGs,[33] although this may be different for presenile AD, where early EEG changes are more likely. So far, various types of quantitative EEG analysis have not been shown to be superior to visual assessment of the EEG in AD.[7,34] Two studies used a simple visual scale, the 'grand total EEG score' or GTE, to assess the value of the EEG in dementia with promising results.[35,36] In the population-based study of Strijers et al, the GTE had a sensitivity of and a specificity comparable to MRI (magnetic resonance imaging) assessment of hippocampal atrophy.[35] The study of Claus et al showed that in cases of diagnostic doubt, an abnormal EEG makes a diagnosis of AD significantly more likely.[36]

The EEG can also be used in the differential diagnosis of AD and other causes of cognitive dysfunction. Depression can be associated with cognitive complaints, but, in contrast to AD, does not give rise to significant EEG abnormalities. According to Jonkman, the total accuracy of the EEG in differentiating between AD and depression with cognitive complaints is between 69% and 84%.[7] AD and toxic metabolic encephalopathy (with delirium) can both give rise to diffuse EEG abnormalities. However, the EEG abnormalities are usually more severe in toxic metabolic encephalopathy. Features such as triphasic waves, epileptiform abnormalities, and FIRDA argue in favor of a metabolic/toxic disorder rather than AD. A simple rule of thumb is the following: 'If the EEG is more affected than the patient, this argues for toxic metabolic encephalopathy; if the patient is more affected than the EEG, this argues for a neurodegenerative disorder such as AD or FTD.' Another frequent clinical problem is the differential diagnosis of AD and vascular dementia. This differentiation is made more difficult by the fact that AD and vascular problems may occur together. The EEG does not allow an absolute distinction between the two, but some EEG features are considered to be suggestive of vascular pathology:

1. asymmetries of physiologic rhythms, in particular the alpha and the mu rhythm
2. focal abnormalities, especially in the temporal regions
3. paroxysmal diffuse abnormalities
4. sharp waves and epileptiform abnormalities.

The EEG in AD may have prognostic as well as diagnostic significance.[37,38] According to Rodriguez et al,[39] EEG changes predict the occurrence of incontinence, loss of activities of daily live, and survival. A loss of beta activity and, to a lesser extent, alpha activity is associated with a less favorable prognosis in AD, even after correction for such factors as disease duration, severity, and age.[40] However, in concluding this section, we should remark that the crucial problem when assessing the value of the EEG in dementia diagnosis is not to determine its sensitivity and specificity, or prognosis, but to find out when and how it may aid in clinical decision-making. We will attempt to address the question later in this chapter.

Other degenerative dementias

As is the case with AD, other neurodegenerative disorders that can give rise to dementia may also be associated with normal EEGs in the early stages. This is especially true for frontotemporal dementia, where the EEG can remain normal quite long although this view has recently been challenged.[41] In an advanced stage, mild abnormalities, usually in the form of low voltage, irregular theta, can be found over the frontal and temporal regions, while the alpha rhythm is still preserved. At the group level, quantitative analysis can aid in differentiating AD from frontotemporal dementia.[42] In supranuclear palsy, the EEG abnormalities are comparable to those in AD. Huntington's disease is often characterized by a so-called 'low voltage' EEG, with an amplitude of the background activity lower than 10 μV. According to Markand,[43] this EEG pattern is rare in healthy subjects, but can be found in 33% of patients with Huntington's disease.

Parkinson's disease is associated with dementia in 20–30% of patients. In non-demented Parkinson patients, the EEG is normal. In demented Parkinson patients, EEG abnormalities can be found with a pattern comparable to AD.[44] When EEG abnormalities do occur in non-demented Parkinson patients, they may have some predictive value for the later occurrence of dementia.[45] A demeting disorder closely related to both AD and Parkinson's disease is dementia with Lewy bodies (DLB). Some authors have suggested that DLB can be differentiated from AD by the occurrence of more severe EEG abnormalities in DLB.[46] However, in a recent large study, no significant EEG differences between AD and DLB could be found.[47] Of interest, in this last study the clinical diagnosis of DLB did not correlate very well with the neuropathologic findings. In fact, there is some doubt as to whether DLB can really be differentiated from Parkinson dementia.

Vascular dementia

Vascular dementia is a somewhat problematic entity because it involves various types of pathology (vascular white matter changes, lacunar infarcts, and multiple cortical infarcts) and their possible relationship with cognitive dysfunction. The basic concept of vascular dementia has three fundamental elements:

1. demonstrated vascular lesions;
2. a dementia syndrome
3. a causal connection between 1 and 2.

In clinical practice, it is often difficult to establish this causal connection with certainty. In the case of two or more large cortical infarcts, the EEG can be expected to show focal abnormalities (focal flattening, slowing, periodic discharges with or without sharp waves, and epileptiform abnormalities); in a more chronic stage, these abnormalities tend to diminish. In the case of diffuse vascular white matter changes, the EEG can show relatively non-specific slowing as well as intermittent temporal slow waves. As indicated in the section on AD, there are some EEG abnormalities that favor vascular pathology over AD:

1. asymmetries of physiologic rhythms, in particular the alpha and the mu rhythm, and asymmetric response on photic stimulation (Farbrot's phenomenon)
2. focal abnormalities, especially in the temporal regions
3. paroxysmal diffuse abnormalities
4. sharp waves and epileptiform abnormalities.

Creutzfeldt–Jakob disease

Creutzfeldt–Jakob disease is a rare cause of dementia, that is, however, important in the present discussion because it is associated with characteristic EEG changes which may have diagnostic significance.[48] The EEG changes depend upon the stage of the disease. In the first phase there are predominantly non-specific abnormalities. There may be a disorganization of the background activity, with an increase in theta and delta activities. In the second stage, the characteristic periodic discharges can be found. These discharges are usually di- or triphasic, last 200–500 ms, and have amplitudes up to 300 μV. The interval between the periodic discharges may vary between 0.5 and 2 seconds. Often the discharges are associated with myoclonic movements, which sometimes have a fixed temporal relation to the discharges. Sometimes the periodic discharges are at first unilateral, and can be classified as PLEDs (periodic lateralized epileptiform discharges). Later in the disease, the discharges usually occur in a bilaterally synchronous fashion, and should be classified as PSIDDs (periodic short-interval diffuse discharges). In the third and final stage of the disease, the PSIDDs persist, and the amplitude of the background activity between the discharges decreases until only the periodic discharges remain.

In general, it can be stated that absence of periodic discharges after a disease duration of 3 months or longer makes a diagnosis of Creutzfeldt–Jakob disease unlikely, but does not exclude it. According to Zerr et al,[49] the periodic discharges have a sensitivity of 66% and a specificity of 74%. The 14-3-3 protein in the liquor has a higher sensitivity and specificity, but the EEG is still considered to be important for the diagnosis.[49] In a recent study involving 206 autopsy confirmed cases, Steinhoff showed that, in subjects with suspected Creutzfeldt–Jakob disease, periodic discharges in the EEG have a sensitivity of 64% and a specificity of 91%.[50]

THE ELECTROENCEPHALOGRAM IN DEMENTIA DIAGNOSIS: A PRACTICAL APPROACH

As became clear in the previous section, the literature on EEG in dementia – only a fraction of which has been reviewed – is somewhat overwhelming, but it is surprisingly difficult to extract practical guidelines from it. In this section, we attempt to give some practical guidelines based on the experience of the Alzheimer Center of the VU University Medical Center in Amsterdam, the Netherlands. At the Alzheimer Center, new patients with cognitive complaints and suspected dementia undergo a 1-day, comprehensive evaluation consisting of a clinical examination, a neuropsychologic examination, blood tests, MRI of the brain, and an EEG recording. All findings are discussed in a multidisciplinary meeting that takes place one and a half weeks later. The multidisciplinary team consists of a neurologist, a psychiatrist, a geriatrician, a nurse, a psychologist, and a clinical neurophysiologist. The findings of the laboratory tests, including the EEG, are discussed in relation to the clinical findings and in relation to each other; a final diagnosis is reached by consensus. In case of doubt, the patient is examined again after 6 months. This approach, where EEG findings are interpreted in relation to other relevant information and not as absolute facts, has proven quite fruitful. The following guidelines are derived from this experience.

When to record an EEG in suspected dementia?

Two strategies can be followed in determining in whom to record EEGs: a selective and a non-selective approach. In the selective approach, advocated for instance by Walstra et al.[51] EEGs are recorded only when the history and clinical examination suggest the presence of a disorder which requires EEG evaluation. This might be the case in suspected epilepsy, toxic metabolic encephalopathy, or Creutzfeldt–Jakob disease. The advantage of this approach is that it makes minimal use of EEG resources, and presumably has a high yield of relevant EEG findings. Alternatively, EEGs can be recorded on a routine basis in all subjects evaluated for dementia. This is the approach followed at the Alzheimer Center. The disadvantage of this approach is that it implies a considerable demand on facilities for recording EEGs. On the other hand, it turns out that the EEG findings that are most interesting, and that have the most pronounced consequences for clinical decisions, are often unexpected. In other words, the EEG can provide relevant information, even in patients in whom a clear indication for recording an EEG on the basis of the history and clinical examination apparently did not exist.

Two examples of unexpected but relevant EEG findings are

- unexpected epileptiform abnormalities;
- frequent apneas, suggestive of obstructive sleep apnea syndrome (OSAS).

Some patients who do not have a clear history of (temporal) epilepsy, and who are not being treated with antiepileptic drugs may present with (temporal) epileptiform abnormalities. This finding has two implications: first, it requires a thorough search for underlying structural abnormalities such as mesiotemporal sclerosis or cortical dysplasia, which may not be obvious on routine MRI; secondly, even if there are no obvious clinical seizures but only memory complaints, treatment with antiepileptic drugs should be considered. In some patients such treatment may actually cure the 'dementia'.[52] Another unexpected but relevant finding is that some patients with cognitive complaints have significant (duration longer than 10 seconds) apneas during the EEG recording. In such patients there is often a pronounced tendency to fall asleep during the recording, and apneas usually appear in non-REM 1. The end of the apnea is usually characterized by an arousal reaction in the EEG. These patients may suffer from OSAS which is known to be associated with cognitive complaints. Also, a relationship between APOE E4 and sleep apnea in AD has been suggested.[53] These patients need to be referred to a specialist sleep center for further diagnosis (24-hour polysomnographic recordings) and treatment.

Other examples of such unexpected relevant EEG findings can be given, but the main point is clear: they will be missed if the EEG is only recorded in selected cases. Because some of the unexpected findings have clear clinical consequences, this argues for recording EEGs in all cases of suspected dementia.

How to record the EEG in dementia?

Recording of the EEG in a patient with cognitive complaints basically follows the same procedure as a routine EEG. There are, however, a few points to be considered. First, some of the provocation tests used in routine recordings such as hyperventilation and photic stimulation are less relevant for the evaluation of dementia, and can be skipped. On the other hand, it may be useful to include a simple cognitive test during the EEG recording, such as serial subtraction of 7 from 100 or a simple memory task. Such a test may provide information on the reactivity of the EEG during cognitive processing, but its use is still a bit experimental.[54] Another issue to be considered is the level of arousal. As indicated before, even slight drowsiness can be associated with an increase in theta activity. Because relative theta power is one of the earliest and most sensitive indicators of early AD, it is extremely important not to confuse drowsiness-related theta activity with pathologic theta activity. During the EEG recording, care should be taken that the patient is well awake during at least part of the recording. On the other hand, it is also useful to allow the patient to fall asleep during another part of the recording, because this may provoke such abnormalities as epileptiform activity and sleep apnea.

How to analyze the EEG?

The cornerstone of clinical EEG is still the visual analysis of the EEG record. This is also true when the EEG is used for the evaluation of dementia. There is no evidence that quantitative analysis is superior to visual assessment. However, visual assessment can be made more accurate and reproducible with the use of simple semiquantitative scales such as the GTE.[35,36] EEG evaluation for dementia should take into account subtle abnormalities, such as minor slowing of the alpha frequency, diminished reactivity, and an increase in low-voltage theta. On the other hand, confusion with normal age-related EEG findings such as BTTE, sleep-onset FIRDA, and SREDA should be avoided. If quantitative analysis is performed, care should be taken that the epochs used for the analysis are not taken from periods with drowsiness, and the results of quantitative analysis should only be used as an adjunct to visual assessment and not as a replacement. Relying solely on sophisticated quantitative analyses of the EEG is courting disaster.[55] Perhaps the most practical approach is to perform a simple frequency analysis and to determine the alpha peak frequency at O_2 and O_1, and the relative theta power at the same electrodes. This simple analysis can be performed with most modern digital EEG machines.

How to interpret the EEG findings?

EEG interpretation involves two different levels. At the first level, the EEG is described without taking into account any other information than the age and level of arousal of the patient. The EEG should be classified as normal or abnormal for age, and, if abnormal, the nature, distribution, and severity of the abnormalities should be indicated, preferably using a semiquantitative scale. At the second level, the EEG findings should be interpreted in the context of the clinical information, but also the findings on other laboratory tests. At this level it is important to consider whether the EEG supports the clinical diagnosis, or suggests alternative possibilities, whether the EEG provides information on prognosis, and whether any unexpected EEG findings may be clinically relevant. The second level of interpretation is obviously the more difficult one, because it requires knowledge of both electroencephalography and the clinical aspects of dementia, but it is indispensable to take full advantage of the contribution of the EEG to the diagnostic process. Assessment of the clinical meaning of the EEG findings can be based upon the clinical information provided by the referring clinician on the EEG form, but the most optimal solution is for the clinical neurophysiologist to take part in the multi-disciplinary team in which all the findings are discussed. As an aid in the clinical interpretation of EEG findings, a schematic overview of the relationship between EEG phenomena and major categories of dementia is given in Table 12.1.

When to repeat the EEG?

Many patients who are referred to memory clinics these days have only mild complaints. Even after extensive evaluation, it is not always possible to make a final diagnosis. Such patients are usually evaluated again after a period of 1 year or 6 months. It is highly recommended to repeat the EEG during such follow-up visits, because this is an objective and sensitive tool to detect slowly progressive brain disease. In particular, slowing of the alpha peak frequency by 1 Hz or more, even when the peak frequency is still within normal limits, is indicative of a progressive encephalopathy. Also when there is doubt about the relative contribution of a toxic metabolic encephalopathy and a degenerative dementia to the condition of a patient, it may be useful to repeat the EEG, because improvement over time argues against a degenerative dementia.

Table 12.1 Electroencephalographic findings in the major categories of dementia

Finding	SMC[a]	AD[b]	FTD[c]	VD[d]	TME[e]	DLB[f]	CJD[g]
Slowing alpha	−−	+	−	0	++	+	+
Diminished reactivity alpha	−−	+	−	0	+	+	+
Asymmetric alpha	−−	−	−−	+	−	−	−
Diff theta	−−	+	−	0	++	+	+
Temporal slow waves	0	0	0	++	0	++	0
Focal abnormalities	−−	−	−	+	−	0	0
Sharp waves	−−	−	−−	+	+	0	0
Periodic discharges	−−	−−	−−	0	+	0	++
FIRDA[h]	−−	−−	−−	0	++	+	0

[a] SMC, subjective memory complaints; the EEG findings in mild cognitive impairment and depression with cognitive dysfunction resemble this pattern.
[b] AD, Alzheimer's disease. Please note that the EEG may be normal in up to 50% with early senile AD, whereas the EEG is often abnormal in presenile AD.
[c] FTD, frontotemporal dementia (there may be a slight increase in frontal low-voltage theta).
[d] VD, vascular dementia. Note that there is often a combination of VD and AD.
[e] TME, toxic metabolic encephalopathy, which often manifests clinically as (silent) delirium.
[f] DLB, dementia with Lewy bodies (closely related to Parkinson dementia).
[g] CJD, Creutzfeldt–Jakob disease.
[h] FIRDA, frontal intermittent rhythmic delta activity.
The prevalence of EEG abnormalities in different dementing disorders is indicated as follows: −− almost never; − infrequently; 0 sometimes; + frequently; ++ almost always.

ELECTROENCEPHALOGRAPHY AND MAGNETOENCEPHALOGRAHY IN DEMENTIA: NEW DEVELOPMENTS AND FUTURE PROSPECTS

The daily practice of EEG in the evaluation of dementia still depends to a large extent upon a straightforward visual analysis of the record, with only minimal support from quantitative analysis. However, there are some interesting developments which may change the way the EEG is used in the evaluation in the near future. These developments fall into two categories:

- development of new sophisticated tools to analyze the EEG
- using magnetoencephalography (MEG) instead of EEG, to record the magnetic fields of the brain.

Today, quantitative analysis of the EEG is still almost synonymous with the use of so-called linear methods such as frequency analysis and coherence analysis. These methods are based upon the assumption that the EEG is essentially a kind of filtered noise. Since the early 1990s, a different approach has been explored. This approach, which is inspired by the theory of non-linear dynamical systems (also called 'chaos theory'), assumes that the brain is a complex, self-organizing network of interacting non-linear dynamical systems.[56] The EEG record reflects the dynamics of these underlying networks, and can be analyzed with new measures such as the correlation dimension,[57] Lyapunov exponents,[58] Kolmogorov entropy,[58] or non-linear measures of synchronization.[59,60] Non-linear analysis of the EEG has suggested that brain dynamics in dementia may be characterized by a loss of complexity, and abnormal functional interactions between brain regions.[61] There are some indications that combining linear and non-linear EEG analysis may improve the diagnostic accuracy of the EEG in dementia.[62,63] However, although this approach holds promise for the future, at this stage it should be considered still experimental.

Another promising new development is the use of MEG instead of EEG to investigate brain function in Alzheimer's disease. MEG has several theoretical advantages over EEG:

- it is hardly disturbed by the conductive properties of the intervening tissues such as the skull
- with modern whole-head systems it is relatively easy to record very large numbers (151 or more) of channels simultaneously
- MEG does not require the use of a reference, which is an advantage in studies of functional connectivity.

In a pilot study, Berendse et al. showed that the MEG in AD is characterized by significant slowing and loss of coherence, not only in the alpha band but essentially in all frequency bands.[64] Temporoparietal slowing of MEG in AD was also demonstrated by Maestu et al.[65] and Fernandez et al.[66] and was found to correlate with hippocampal atrophy.[67,68] Combining non-linear analysis with MEG further extends the scope of functional studies in AD. Using two different measures of brain complexity, van Cappellen showed that complexity loss in AD depends upon the frequency bands analyzed.[69] Synchronization likelihood analysis of MEG in early AD patients showed a loss of synchronization in the upper alpha, the beta, and the gamma band.[70] In this study, non-linear analysis proved to be more sensitive than coherence analysis. MEG may also be useful in discriminating subjects with mild cognitive impairment, which can be an early stage of Alzheimer's disease, from healthy controls.[71] In conclusion, the use of MEG in the evaluation of dementia holds many promises. However, future clinical application will depend upon replication of the results from pilot studies, and a wider availability of whole-head MEG recording systems in clinical settings.

REFERENCES

1. Wallin A, Brun A, Gustafson L. Swedish consensus on dementia disease. Acta Neurol Scand 1994;Suppl 157:3–31.

2. Knopman DS, DeKosky ST, Cummings JL, et al. Practice parameter: diagnosis of dementia (an evidence-based review). Report of the Quality Standards Subcommittee of the American Academy of Neurology. Neurology 2001;56:1143–1153.

3. Klass DW, Brenner RP. Electro-encephalography of the elderly. J Clin Neurophysiol 1995;12:116–131.

4. Soininen H, Partanen J, Laulumaa V, et al. Longitudinal EEG spectral analysis in early stage of Alzheimer's disease. Electroencephalogr Clin Neurophysiol 1989;72:290–297.

5. Brenner RP. EEG in convulsive and nonconvulsive status epilepticus. J Clin Neurophysiol 2004;21:319–333.

6. Boerman RH, Scheltens P, Weinstein HC. Clinical neurophysiology in the diagnosis of Alzheimer's disease. Clin Neurol Neurosurg 1994;96:111–118.

7. Jonkman EJ. The role of the electro-encephalogram in the diagnosis of dementia of the Alzheimer type: an attempt at technology assessment.

Neurophysiol Clin 1997;27:211–219.

8. Jeong J. EEG dynamics in patients with Alzheimer's disease. Clin Neurophysiol 2004;115:1490–1505.

9. Delbeuck X, Van der Linder M, Colette F. Alzheimer's disease as a disconnection syndrome? Neuropsychol Rev 2003;13:79–92.

10. Nunez PL, Srinivasan R, Westdorp AF, et al. EEG coherency. I: Statistics, reference electrode, volume conduction, Laplacians, cortical imaging, and interpretation at multiple scales. Electroencephalogr Clin Neurophysiol 1997;103:499–515.

11. Leuchter AF, Newton TF, Cook AA, Walter DO. Changes in brain functional connectivity in Alzheimer-type and multi-infarct dementia. Brain 1992;115(Pt 5):1543–1561.

12. Besthorn C, Forstl H, Geiger-Kabisch C, et al. EEG coherence in Alzheimer disease. Electroencephalogr Clin Neurophysiol 1994;90:242–245.

13. Dunkin JJ, Leuchter AF, Newton TF, Cook IA. Reduced EEG coherence in dementia: state or trait marker? Biol Psychiatry 1994;35:870–879.

14. Jelic V, Shigeta M, Julin P, et al. Quantitative electroencephalography

power and coherence in Alzheimer's disease and mild cognitive impairment. Dementia 1996;7:314–323.

15. Locatelli T, Cursi M, Liberati D, Francheschi M, Comi G. EEG coherence in Alzheimer's disease. Electroencephalogr Clin Neurophysiol 1998;106:229–237

16. Knott V, Mohr E, Mahoney C, Ilivitsky V. Electroencephalographic coherence in Alzheimer's disease: comparisons with a control group and population norms. J Geriatr Psychiatry Neurol 2000;13:1–8.

17. Stevens A, Kircher T, Nickola M, et al. Dynamic regulation of EEG power and coherence is lost early and globally in probable DAT. Eur Arch Psychiatry Clin Neurosci 2001; 251:199–204.

18. Adler G, Brassen S, Jajcevic A. EEG coherence in Alzheimer's dementia. J Neural Transm 2003;110:1051–1058.

19. Hogan MJ, Swanwick GRJ, Kaiser J, Rowan M, Lawlor B. Memory-related EEG power and coherence reductions in mild Alzheimer's disease. Int J Psychophysiol 2003;49:147–163.

20. Babiloni C, Miniussi C, Moretti DV, et al. Cortical networks generating movement-related EEG rhythms in Alzheimer's disease: an EEG coherence study. Behav Neurosci 2004; 118:698–706.

21. Koenig T, Prichep L, Dierks T, et al. Decreased EEG synchronization in Alzheimer's disease and mild cognitive impairment. Neurobiol Aging 2005;26:165–171.

22. Riekkinen P, Buzsaki G, Riekkinen P Jr, Soininen H, Partanen J. The cholinergic system and EEG slow waves. Electroencephalogr Clin Neurophysiol 1991;78:89–96.

23. Francis PT, Palmer AM, Snape M, Wilcock GK. The cholinergic hypothesis of Alzheimer's disease: a review of the progress. J Neurol Neurosurg Psychiatry 1999;66: 137–147.

24. Shigeta M, Persson A, Viitanen M, Winblad B, Nordberg A. EEG regional changes during long-term treatment with tetrahydroaminoacridine (THA) in Alzheimer's disease. Acta Neurol Scand Suppl 1993;149:58–61.

25. Adler G, Brassen S. Short-term rivastigmine treatment reduces EEG slow-wave power in Alzheimer patients. Neuropsychobiology 2001; 43:273–276

26. Adler G, Brassen S, Chwalek K, Dieter B, Teufel M. Prediction of treatment response to rivastigmine in Alzheimer's dementia. J Neurol Neurosurg Psychiatry 2004;75:292–294.

27. Ricceri L, Minghetti L, Moles A, et al. Cognitive and neurological deficits induced by early and prolonged basal forebrain cholinergic hypofunction in rats. Exp Neurol 2004;189:162–172.

28. Villa AEP, Tetko IV, Dutoit P, Vantini G. Non-linear cortico-cortical interactions modulated by cholinergic afferences from the rat basal forebrain. BioSystems 2000;58:219–228.

29. Stern EA, Bacskai BJ, Hickey GA, et al. Cortical synaptic integration in vivo is disrupted by amyloid-plaques. J Neurosci 2004;24:4535–4540.

30. Lehtovirta M, Partanen J, Kononen M, et al. Spectral analysis of EEG in Alzheimer's disease: relation to apolipoprotein E polymorphism. Neurobiol Aging 1996;4:523–526.

31. Jelic V, Julin P, Shigeta M et al. Apolipoprotein E ε4 allele decreases functional connectivity in Alzheimer's disease as measured by EEG coherence. J Neurol Neurosurg Psychiatry 1997;63:59–65.

32. Prinz PN, Larsen LH, Moe KE, Vitiello MV. EEG markers of early Alzheimer's disease in computer selected tonic REM sleep. Electroencephalogr Clin Neurophysiol 1992;83:36–43.

33. Soininen H, Riekkinen PJ Sr. EEG in diagnostics and follow-up of

Alzheimer's disease. Acta Neurol Scand Suppl 1992;139:36–39.

34. Brenner R, Reynolds III ChF, Ulrich RF. Diagnostic efficacy of computerized spectral versus visual EEG analysis in elderly normal, demented and depressed subjects. Electroencephalogr Clin Neurophysiol 1988; 69:110–117.

35. Strijers RL, Scheltens Ph, Jonkman EJ, et al. Diagnosing Alzheimer's disease in community-dwelling elderly: a comparison of EEG and MRI. Dement Geratr Cogn Disord 1997;8:198–202.

36. Claus JJ, Strijers RLM, Jonkman EJ, et al. The diagnostic value of electroencephalography in mild senile Alzheimer's disease. Clin Neurophysiol 1999;110:825–832.

37. Helkala EL, Laulumaa V, Soininen H, Partanen J, Riekkinen PJ. Different patterns of cognitive decline related to normal or deteriorating EEG in a 3-year follow-up study of patients with Alzheimer's disease. Neurology 1991;41:528–532.

38. Lopez OL, Brenner RP, Becker JT, et al. EEG spectral abnormalities and psychosis as predictors of cognitive and functional decline in probable Alzheimer's disease. Neurology 1997; 48:1521–1525.

39. Rodriguez G, Nobili F, Arrigo A, et al. Prognostic significance of quantitative electroencephalography in Alzheimer patients: preliminary observations. Electroencephalogr Clin Neurophysiol 1996;99:123–128.

40. Claus JJ, Ongerboer de Visser BW, Walstra GJM, et al. Quantitative spectral electroencephalography in predicting survival in patients with early Alzheimer disease. Arch Neurol 1998; 55:1105–1111.

41. Chan D, Walters RJ, Sampson EL, et al. EEG abnormalities in frontotemporal lobar degeneration. Neurology 2004;62:1628–1630.

42. Yener GG, Leuchter AF, Jenden D, et al. Quantitative EEG in frontotemporal dementia. Clin Electroencephalogr 1996;27:61–68.

43. Markand ON. Organic brain syndromes and dementias. In: Daly DD, Pedley TA, eds. Current Practice of Clinical Electroencephalography, 2nd edn. New York: Raven Press, 1990.

44. Neufeld MY, Inzelberg R, Korczyn AD. EEG in demented and non-demented Parkinsonian patients. Acta Neurol Scand 1988,78:1–5.

45. de Weerd AW, Perquin WVM, Jonkman EJ. Role of the EEG in the prediction of dementia in Parkinson's disease. Dementia 1990;1:115–118.

46. Briel RCG, McKeith IG, Barker WA, et al. EEG findings in dementia with Lewy bodies and Alzheimer's disease. J Neurol Neurosurg Psychiatry 1999; 66:401–403.

47. Londos E, Passant U, Brun A, et al. Regional cerebral blood flow and EEG in clinically diagnosed dementia with Lewy bodies and Alzheimer's disease. Arch Gerontol Geriatr 2003:36: 231–245.

48. Steinhoff BJ, Racker S, Herrendorf G, et al. Accuracy and reliability of periodic sharp wave complexes in Creutzfeldt–Jakob disease. Arch Neurol 1996;53:162–166.

49. Zerr I, Pocchiari M, Collins S, et al. Analysis of EEG and CSF 14-3-3 proteins as aids to the diagnosis of Creutzfeldt–Jakob disease. Neurology 2000;55:811–815.

50. Steinhoff BJ, Zerr I, Glatting M, et al. Diagnostic value of periodic complexes in Creutzfeldt–Jakob disease. Ann Neurol 2004;56:702–708.

51. Walstra GJ, Teunisse S, van Gool WA, van Crevel H. Reversible dementia in elderly patients referred to a memory clinic. J Neurol 1997;244:17–22.

52. Hogh P, Smith SJ, Scahill RI, et al. Epilepsy presenting as AD: neuroimaging, electrical features, and response to treatment. Neurology 2002;58:298–301.

53. Bliwise DL. Sleep apnea, APOE4 and Alzheimer's disease. 20 years and counting? J Psychosom Res 2002; 53:539–546.

54. Pijnenburg YAL, van de Made Y, van Cappellen van Walsum AM, et al. EEG synchronization likelihood in mild cognitive impairment and Alzheimer's disease during a working memory task. Clin Neurophysiol 2004;115:1332–1339.

55. Nuwer MR, Nauser HM. Erroneous diagnosis using EEG discriminant analysis. Neurology 1994;44:1998–2000.

56. Stam CJ. Chaos, continuous EEG, and cognitive mechanisms: a future for clinical neurophysiology. Am J END Technol 2003;43:1–17.

57. Pritchard WS, Duke DW, Coburn KL. Altered EEG dynamical responsivity associated with normal aging and probable Alzheimer's disease. Dementia 1991;2: 102–105.

58. Stam CJ, Jelles B, Achtereekte HAM, et al. Investigation of EEG non-linearity in dementia and Parkinson's disease. Electroencephalogr Clin Neurophysiol 1995;95:309–317.

59. Jeong J, Gore JC, Peterson BS. Mutual information analysis of the EEG in patients with Alzheimer's disease. Clin Neurophysiol 2001; 112:827–835.

60. Stam CJ, van der Made Y, Pijnenburg YAL, Scheltens Ph. EEG synchronization in mild cognitive impairment and Alzheimer's disease. Acta Neurol Scand 2003;108:90–96.

61. Jeong J. Nonlinear dynamics of EEG in Alzheimer's disease. Drug Dev Res 2002;56:57–66.

62. Pritchard WS, Duke DW, Coburn KL, et al. EEG-based, neural-net predictive classification of Alzheimer's disease versus control subjects is augmented by non-linear EEG measures. Electroencephalogr Clin Neurophysiol 1994,91:118–130.

63. Stam CJ, Jelles B, Achtereekte HAM, van Birgelen JH, Slaets JPJ. Diagnostic usefulness of linear and nonlinear quantitative EEG analysis in Alzheimer's disease. Clin Electroencephalogr 1996;27:69–77.

64. Berendse HW, Verbunt JPA, Scheltens Ph, van Dijk BW, Jonkman EJ. Magnetoencephalographic analysis of cortical activity in Alzheimer's disease. A pilot study. Clin Neurophysiol 2000;111:604–612.

65. Maestu F, Fernandez A, Simos PG, et al. Spatio-temporal patterns of brain magnetic activity during a memory task in Alzheimer's disease. Neuroreport 2001;12:3917–3922.

66. Fernandez A, Maestu F, Amo C, et al. Focal temporoparietal slow activity in Alzheimer's disease revealed by magnetoencephalography. Biol Psychiatry 2002;52:764–770.

67. Fernandez A, Arazzola J, Maestu F, et al. Correlations of hippocampal atrophy and focal low-frequency magnetic activity in Alzheimer disease: volumetric MR imaging – magnetoencephalographic study. AJNR Am J Neuroradiol 2003;24:481–487.

68. Maestu F, Arrazola J, Fernandez A et al. Do cognitive patterns of brain magnetic activity correlate with hippocampal atrophy in Alzheimer's disease? J Neurol Neurosurg Psychiatry 2003;74:208–212.

69. van Cappellen van Walsum AM, Pijnenburg YAL, Berendse HW, et al. A neural complexity measure applied to MEG data in Alzheimer's disease. Clin Neurophysiology 2003;114: 1034–1040.

70. Stam CJ, van Cappellen van Walsum AM, Pijnenburg YAL, et al. Generalized synchronization of MEG recordings in Alzheimer's disease: evidence for involvement of the gamma band. J Clin Neurophysiol 2002;19:562–574.

71. Puregger E, Walla P, Deecke L, Dal-Bianco P. Magnetoencephalographic features related to mild cognitive impairment. Neuroimage 2003;20:2235–2244.

Index

Numbers in *italics* refer to tables and figures.